Advance prais
Diabetic

MW00800350

"*Diabetic Eye Disease: Lessons From A Diabetic Eye Doctor* is one of the most down to earth and practical books on this topic ever written. It takes a complicated subject and explains things in clear black and white terms and leaves no doubt in the reader's mind. This book will undoubtedly help the many people living with diabetes and eye disease and those hoping to avoid it."

--Steven V. Edelman, M.D.
UC San Diego School of Medicine,
Division of Diabetes & Metabolism
Founder & Director, *Taking Control of Your Diabetes*

"Dr. Paul Chous has done a wonderful job of describing diabetic eye disease and the current thoughts on management, in a way that is understandable and engaging for people of all backgrounds. This book is a welcome addition for all patients to have a better understanding of their disease. Thank goodness Dr. Chous has written such a thoughtful work.

--William K.M. Shields, M.D.
Retina & Macula Specialists
Renton, Tacoma and Olympia, Washington

"It is very timely to have a book written by a doctor who has diabetes himself and who can communicate so effectively with patients who have diabetes. This book is clearly written, easy to understand, with a message that gives all diabetic patients hope. I recommend it for anyone with diabetes, the lay public and doctors too!"

--Lesley L. Walls, O.D., M.D.
Professor/Family Practice Physician
President, *Southern California College of Optometry*

"It's a thrill to discover a great book about diabetes. Its a thrill that is all too rare...I will add it to my list of a baker's dozen books that I think are worth the attention of most anyone with diabetes...this new book zeros in on one of the worst complications of the disease: diabetic eye disease. In fact, there is nothing in the published literature that comes close to what Dr. A. Paul Chous offers us."

--Rick Mendosa
Free Lance Health Writer on the Web
Publisher, *Diabetes Update Newsletter*

Diabetic Eye Disease

Lessons From a *Diabetic* Eye Doctor

How to Avoid Blindness and Get *Great* Eye Care

A. Paul Chous, M.A., O.D.

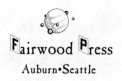

Fairwood Press

Auburn•Seattle

Diabetic Eye Disease

A Fairwood Press Book
April 2003
Copyright © 2003 by A. Paul Chous

All Rights Reserved

No part of this book may be reproduced or transmitted in any form or
by any means, electronic or mechanical, including photocopying, recording,
or by any information storage and retrieval system, without
permission in writing from the publisher.

Fairwood Press
5203 Quincy Ave SE
Auburn, WA   98092
www.fairwoodpress.com

Cover art © Getty Images/The Image Bank
Cover and Book Design by Patrick Swenson

ISBN: 0-9668184-7-4
First Fairwood Press Edition: April 2003
Printed in the United States of America

Diabetic
Eye Disease

Dedication

For the great teachers, mentors and inspirations of my life: my dad and mom, Charlie and Alice Chous; my brother, Dr. Robert Chous; Professor Creel Froman of the *University of California at Irv*ine; my long-time friend and exemplar of taking the road less traveled, Mark Evans of *Associated Press*; Elizabeth, Atticus, and my best friend, Pete. I could not be who I am without them.

Acknowledgements

I would like to acknowledge the doctors of *Pacific Cataract and Laser Institute* for their assistance with photographs, and William K.M. Shields, M.D. for his suggestions and support. Much appreciation is due to my own endocrinologist, K. David McCowen, M.D., who has given me the finest care and always been on my side. Thanks also to all my diabetic patients and their families who have taught me more than they know.

Finally, thanks to my friends and colleagues of the UC Berkeley School of Optometry *Class of 1991*, who I am fortunate enough to spend time with camping each and every year since 1988: Drs. Bruce Abramson, Ron Black, Brent Chinn, Ron Garcia, Greg Hom, Chris Kavanagh, Dave Redman, Rand Siekert, Tony Soria, Bob Theaker, Kevin Tsuda and Rick Vanover. These fine gentlemen have not only made me a better doctor, but have helped me realize the essential meaning and importance of friendship.

Disclaimer

The information and recommendations contained in this publication are generally consistent with the medical and optometric standards of care for patients with diabetes, but also reflect the author's experience and opinions. All reasonable steps have been taken to ensure the accuracy of information presented. However, the author and publisher cannot ensure the efficacy or safety of any product or service described herein for all patients. Individuals are advised to consult a physician or other appropriate health care professionals before undertaking any diet, exercise or medication regimen referred to in this publication. The author, publisher and their agents assume no responsibility or liability for personal or other injury, loss, or damage that may result from recommendations or information in this publication.

Contents

Chapter One:

Lessons From A
Diabetic Eye Doctor

Diabetes is currently an incurable disease, which means that every person diagnosed with diabetes has to "deal" with it for the rest of her or his life. Although good medical treatment is widely available and is, in many cases, life saving, the underlying disorder remains. Even those Type 1 diabetics (commonly called *insulin dependant* or *juvenile-onset*) who have received pancreas (or islet cell) transplants, a seeming cure, must face the threat of immune system destruction and/or rejection of transplanted tissue. The genetic triggers that caused diabetes by allowing the immune system to attack the pancreas are always there. Even Type 2 diabetics (also commonly known as *adult-onset* or *non-insulin dependent*) who achieve normal blood sugar levels with diet and exercise, and without the use of medication, still have diabetes. **Diabetes does not just "go away."** A person may have borderline hyperglycemia (also known as *impaired glucose tolerance* or *pre-diabetes*), but once the clinical definition and specific criteria for diabetes have been met, the person in question has diabetes — period. **There is no such animal as "borderline diabetes." Like pregnancy, you either have it or you don't.**

Given that a diagnosis of diabetes has been made, the most important question is, **"How will you deal with your condition?"** This sounds like a simple question, but really it is not. In fact, there are many ways of dealing with diabetes, some of which are more or less beneficial and some of which are more or less detrimental. Moreover, some strategies will work better for some diabetics than others, some will work only at certain times during one's life (based upon both physiology and emotional state), and some clinically proven strategies will not work for certain diabetics at all. ***This is not to say that there are no fundamental principles of good diabetes management — there are, and much of this book is devoted to explaining them.*** **It is to say that there is more than one path to managing diabetes well, and that finding the right strategies for any particular person must be done on an individualized, life-long basis.**

Finding the right strategy takes time, patience, determination and, most importantly, *education*. It is the author's hope that this book will serve to make diabetic patients, their families and their friends more aware of the fundamental principles of good diabetes management in general, and of the specific eye complications caused by diabetes, and their relationship to good diabetes management, in particular. Armed with this information, patients and their advocates will be better able to develop reasonable strategies for "dealing with" diabetes and avoiding *complications* in the eyes or other parts of the body.

What is "Good" Diabetes Management?

Good diabetes management covers the span of an individual's diabetic life (from the time of diagnosis forward) but consists of a series of management decisions, treatments and goals that *change* **as a person's body changes (both due to the normal aging process and the development of complications), as new treatments become available, and as new strategies for improved control are learned.** ***This point cannot be stressed enough.*** Like most chronic health conditions, there is no "magic bullet" for diabetes control. No "system" works perfectly forever, and strategies must often change to keep up with changes in one's health status. **With advances in medical knowledge and biotechnology, the "gold standards" of today will undoubtedly become antiquated and sub-standard in the future.** The history of medical science is filled with examples of this phenomenon.

What does "good diabetes management" mean? Foregoing medical jargon for now, a reasonable definition might be: **"controlling diabetes in such a way that the person in question is able to experience life in the fullest way possible without insurmountable physical disability caused by diabetes and with a minimum of emotional stress."**

Put more simply, good diabetes management means a patient suffers the dreaded complications of diabetes to the smallest degree possible with the least hassle possible. It does not necessarily mean patients will have <u>no</u> complications (although that is certainly a worthy goal), only that those complications, if they occur, will not prevent patients from reaching their life goals or maximizing their unique human abilities.

Controlling diabetes effectively is an individualized effort, but it should not be an individual one. Controlling diabetes should be a team effort amongst the patient, family and closest friends, and a *team of health care professionals who are knowledgeable about and keenly interested in diabetes*. I am intimately familiar with several different strategies for controlling diabetes, both as a Type 1 diabetic for 34 years, and as a doctor of optometry managing the eye complications of diabetes for the last twelve years. I have managed my own condition differently at different points in my life, and I have seen several thousand of my own diabetic patients manage their conditions using a variety of different strategies. Some diabetics ignore their disease, living life exactly as they did prior to diagnosis. Others meticulously monitor their blood sugars, medications and diets, frequently consult with health care professionals to check for the earliest signs of diabetes complications, read many journal articles describing all the latest diabetes research, and attend lectures on every aspect of diabetes management. Most diabetics probably fall somewhere between these two extremes. Somewhere in between is where I started 34 years ago.

My Story

I was diagnosed with diabetes just after my fifth birthday. My life changed immediately as I required daily injections of insulin, faced numerous episodes of extremely high and low blood sugars (the latter of which sent me to the hospital on four occasions within two years of being diagnosed), and found my parents' and older brother's lives increasingly focused on "protecting" me. In those first years of living with my diabetes, I never thought much about how I was dealing with my condition, as the changes in my life were thrust upon me and seemed dramatic enough to constitute a strategy of sorts. My family helped me to do what the doctor recommended, performing urinalysis twice daily, taking a sizeable injection of pork insulin each morning (with the help of my dad until age seven, when I started to self-inject), measuring my meal portions carefully and avoiding foods containing refined sugar, and exercising regularly (as kids of my age and pre-computer generation were prone to do). In large measure, this represented the gold standard of diabetes management in 1968.

I began to visit a diabetes specialist, an endocrinologist, at age eleven. He changed my insulin regimen a bit, recommended that I start using the newly available, color-coded blood glucose test strips in addition to testing for urine glucose, briefly touched on the various long-term complications associated with diabetes, and suggested that I attend a support group for diabetic children that would allow me to share and discuss my experiences. I rejected the last suggestion outright, and I remember quite vividly telling him that "I am an individual, and do not want to be thrown together with a bunch of diabetic kids any more than you would want to belong to a group of people simply because they have gray hair like you do!" My mom was mortified by the remark, but my conviction that day marked a turning point in the way I was dealing with my diabetes, in my management strategy.

I was on the verge of becoming a teenager and, like most teenagers, yearned to find my individuality and my autonomy. I did not want to be seen as just another diabetic. I began to develop a firm determination that diabetes would play as small a role in my life as possible. I continued taking my shots of insulin, but paid less and less attention to the other details. I felt quite well most of the time. As every diabetic can attest, high blood sugar (hyperglycemia) has little impact upon one's ability to function until it becomes extreme, and although low blood sugar (hypoglycemia) is disabling, it can be corrected quickly or avoided altogether by keeping the blood sugar at least "a little high." I noticed that I felt just as well with moderate hyperglycemia as I did with normal blood sugar levels. I noticed that I felt the same whether or not I even checked my blood sugars, or whether or not I saw the endocrinologist regularly. My annual visits to the foot doctor and eye doctor were always normal, so there seemed to be no problem with my strategy.

By the time I entered college, the attention I paid to my diabetes was truly minimal. My diet consisted mostly of high fat foods and non-complex carbohydrates (more on this later). I exercised regularly and felt quite well, taking insulin injections before each meal (a strategy I adopted on my own that allowed me to eat whenever I chose without the risk of hypoglycemia posed by less frequent injections of long acting insulin), and rarely checking my blood glucose levels. I developed a lot of confidence in my ability to gauge my blood sugar levels by the way I felt, rather than by actually *measuring* my blood sugar (a confidence which, as I will explain later, was completely erroneous and unjustified). At the start of my senior year, I visited my optometrist who told me I had the beginning stages of diabetic retinopathy and should try to take better control of my blood sugars. He asked to see me again in six months for a recheck. As I had never felt better in my life, and my eyesight on the eye chart test was excellent, his advice went in one ear and out the other, so to speak.

Prior to starting graduate school, I saw a retinal specialist located next door to my endocrinologist's office. In the back of my mind, I thought about what the optometrist had told me the year before. Before leaving town, I wanted to get a clean bill of health and had been encouraged by my older brother, a third year optometry student, to see a specialist. I was still able to see the bottom row on the eye chart, and was more than confident that my eyes were perfect. However, after dilating my eyes, the doctor informed me that I had a lot of internal bleeding, as well as abnormal blood vessel growth on the surface of my retinas. He said my eyes were "like a time bomb, waiting to go off." Like the year before, I again was incredulous. How could my condition be so serious without any symptoms? He photographed the inside of my eyes to show me what he saw, and to explain its significance. I listened, but grasped little of what he was saying, like a lot of patients when they are first told there is something seriously wrong with their health. The doctor scheduled an appointment for laser treatment the next morning. I was supposed to leave for Berkeley the next day, where I was starting a Master's degree program. I decided that laser treatment would have to wait.

As I packed my things that night in preparation for a long road trip, my brother phoned me at home to talk. I shared with him what the optometrist had told me a year earlier, and what the retinal specialist had said that day. I explained that I had no symptoms at all, and that I didn't see the need for laser treatment right away, that it would have to wait until winter or spring. My brother listened patiently, and then repeated much of what both the optometrist and the retinal specialist had already told me about diabetic retinopathy: how it is the leading cause of blindness in young persons, how it may cause no symptoms until irreparable eye damage has occurred, and how laser treatment reduces the risk of vision loss. I began to cry, but he continued, saying that he was concerned that I might not see the retinal specialist for treatment, and he wanted to stress how important it was that I keep my appointment. He said that I was in "serious trouble," and that he would help me in any way he could but, first, I would have to help myself by keeping my appointment. I agreed that I would.

The next morning I saw the specialist, who informed me that I had severe "proliferative diabetic retinopathy" and would require immediate laser treatment. I explained to him that I was a poor college student, without medical insurance, and that I wasn't sure how I could afford his services. He agreed to let me pay in monthly installments of whatever I could afford, and led me to the laser room. My brother held my hand while the laser treatment was performed. As I left the exam room, the specialist remarked that my brother's words had probably saved my sight. Knowing what I know now, I am sure he was right.

Six years and four laser treatments later, I graduated from the UC Berkeley School of Optometry, where I spent a great deal of time learning about the effects of diabetes on the eyes. In clinical externships at three major medical centers, I saw these effects firsthand and discovered quickly that retinopathy was only one of several eye diseases frequently seen in diabetic patients. After spending so much time in the eye doctor's office, and having my life so profoundly affected by my eye doctors, I decided that I wanted to be an eye doctor and work diligently to reduce the eye complications of diabetes. I went into private practice and began explaining my story to every diabetic patient that I met. Soon, I was seeing more and more diabetic patients, was reading more and more books, journal articles and research papers on diabetes, was speaking at hospitals and clinics and health fairs about diabetes and the eye, and was asked to be a consultant to the *American Diabetes Association*. I began to be interviewed by local radio and television stations, and was writing articles for print media.

In 1992, I began seeing an outstanding endocrinologist in Tacoma, Washington. He taught me more about the medical management of my diabetes than any doctor I had seen before, and helped me to achieve the best blood sugar control of my entire diabetic life, as well as stave off the beginning stages of diabetic kidney disease. I began taking multiple home blood glucose measurements each and every day, combining this data with a sliding scale insulin regimen to optimize my blood sugars, especially as revealed by my quarterly glycosylated hemoglobin readings (more on this critically important test later). I began treatment with a so-called "angiotensin conversion enzyme inhibitor" (*ACE inhibitor* for short) which actually reversed my diabetic kidney disease. I watched my diet closely, eating foods with a low "glycemic index" whenever possible, and began exercising regularly.

In 1998, the *American Diabetes Association* presented me with its distinguished "Public Service Award" for my efforts to organize and administer a diabetic eye disease screening campaign aimed at reaching under served diabetic patients, particularly Native, African and Hispanic Americans. Before the birth of my son in 2000, my wife, also a doctor of optometry, developed gestational diabetes that required insulin injections and very tight blood sugar control; as I said to her at the time, at least she married the most sympathetic of guys. In 2002, I began a clinical research project to investigate the accuracy of diabetic patients' abilities to predict their own blood sugars, and began preparing to take the "Certified Diabetes Educator" examination, hoping to become one of the first optometrists to receive this credential.

The evolution of my strategies for managing my diabetes has not been easy, and there have been many setbacks along the way. I still have some high blood glucose readings due to over-indulgence, forgetfulness, illnesses like the occasional cold or flu, poor planning, stress and the vagaries of human existence. I very nearly lost my eyesight and was heading toward kidney failure, so my lifelong diabetes management strategy certainly has been no paragon of virtue. Of course, I will have to continue managing my diabetes for the rest of my life, or until a definitive cure is found.

Happily, though, my strategy for "dealing" with diabetes has been transformed completely over the last 35 years. I have gone from a position of (now) totally antiquated management to one of almost total indifference (as well as imminent medical disaster), and then to a position of being proactive through tight blood sugar control, frequent follow-ups with my team of doctors, and ever-increasing knowledge in my efforts to become the best educated patient and eye doctor possible. It is this last facet of my strategy, I believe, that is the most important to *living a high quality life in spite of diabetes: the willingness to investigate, learn and adapt.* Medical science continues to make advances, and the research of tomorrow will, no doubt, make at least parts of my current strategy obsolete. **To be a good strategy, any strategy for managing diabetes must remain a "work in progress."**

I have been giving talks on diabetic eye disease and principles of good diabetes management to patients throughout Western Washington State for the last ten years, mostly in small group settings at community clinics, diabetes support group meetings and individual doctors' offices. I am both pleased and astonished by how often patients tell me they appreciate my taking the time to explain exactly how and why diabetes causes eye complications, and why good diabetes control is so important; many say they are hearing this information for the first time. I am pleased because it means that I am fulfilling, at least in part, my professional mission to help diabetic patients and their families. I am astonished because much of this information is well known within the general community of health care professionals, is vitally important to helping patients commit to good diabetes management, and should be shared by these patients' own doctors on a regular basis.

Doctors are, of course, busy people who are responsible for seeing large numbers of patients, and their time with individual patients often is limited. All good doctors want what is best for their patients, and in the current health care environment, this can mean making medical recommendations and prescribing treatments by edict, without fully explaining the rationale behind them or engaging patients to take an active role in their own treatment. While this approach may work nicely for acute illnesses requiring short-term treatment (for example, antibiotics prescribed for a common bacterial infection), it does not work well at all for chronic medical conditions, like diabetes, where patients need to take an active, participatory role in the successful management of their condition. Patients live with diabetes, and must control it through their own actions, every minute of every day. It makes absolute sense that patients be empowered to take control of their diabetes through medical education, understanding and encouragement. And so I have written this book, in hope that my experiences, both as a long time diabetic and an eye doctor passionately interested in diabetes, may help you or someone you love to positively transform the way you manage diabetes.

Key Points

1. There are many different strategies for living with diabetes. Finding the right one involves experience, consultation with knowledgeable health care professionals, and education.

2. A good strategy is a "work in progress," changing as medical knowledge advances, as patients learn more, and as their bodies change over time.

3. Good diabetes management means preventing complications to the greatest extent possible while living your life to the fullest.

Section One:

The Fundamentals of Diabetes

Chapter Two:

The Epidemiology of Diabetes and Its Complications

Before delving into the ways in which diabetes causes complications, with a particular emphasis on eye complications, it will be useful to review the *"epidemiology"* of diabetes and its complications; that is, the "statistics" or "numbers" that demonstrate the impact diabetes currently has on the health of the population, as well as the financial burden diabetes places on the economy. It is important to remember that epidemiology reflects the effects of various diseases on the well being of *entire populations*, but that these statistics represent real people and their families who must face the potentially tragic consequences of these diseases.

Diabetes currently affects more than 17 million Americans, of which number the *American Diabetes Association* estimates 5 million have not yet been diagnosed. One and one-half million (8.8%) have Type 1 diabetes, which is also known as "Insulin Dependant Diabetes Mellitus" (IDDM) or "juvenile diabetes," as most (but not all) Type 1 patients are diagnosed before adulthood. Sixteen million Americans (90.2%) have Type 2 diabetes, also called "Non-insulin Dependent Diabetes Mellitus" (NIDDM) or "adult onset diabetes," as most (but not all) Type 2 patients are diagnosed in adulthood. A small number of people (less than 1%) get diabetes as a result of specific genetic defects, medications, tumors and other diseases.

While diabetes affects males and females of all ages and racial groups, some populations have a higher risk: African-Americans and Hispanic-Americans have about twice the risk compared to the general population; Native Americans and Americans of Pacific Island descent have roughly two and one half times the risk compared to the general population. It is believed that these unequal risks result from a combination of genetic and environmental factors, though greater weight most probably rests with the latter.

Type 2 Diabetes – An American Epidemic

The **incidence** of Type 2 diabetes has increased 44% in the last ten years ("incidence" is defined as the number of *new cases in a year's time*), with a 6% growth per year in the **prevalence** of Type 2 diabetes ("prevalence" is defined as the *total number* of patients having the condition). Much of this increase is thought to be directly attributable to an increase in the prevalence of obesity in the United States. Interestingly, the prevalence of Type 2 diabetes amongst juveniles has grown at alarming rates over the last three decades; in fact, children with Type 2 diabetes are the fastest growing subpopulation of diabetics based on percentage growth of this group (1110% growth from 1967 through 1998). Most experts believe this is due to an increase in excess caloric intake (i.e. too much high fat, high carbohydrate, high calorie food) as well as childhood obesity, factors known to be associated with the development of Type 2 diabetes. Even so, the great majority of Type 2 patients are adults, the prevalence increasing with advancing age so that **18% of all Americans past the age of 65 have Type 2 diabetes**. Approximately 800,000 new cases of diabetes are diagnosed each year in the US (2,400 per day).

The Dreaded Complications:
What You Need To Know

Diabetes is the leading cause of kidney failure and renal dialysis, the leading cause of non-traumatic amputation, the leading cause of new cases of blindness and severe vision loss for people under the age of 74, and the sixth leading cause of death overall in the United States. Approximately 100,000 Americans per year experience renal failure from diabetes. Diabetes accounts for roughly 32,000 toe amputations, 12,000 foot amputations and 36,000 leg amputations per year in the US. Between twenty and twenty five thousand Americans are blinded by diabetes each year. Cardiovascular (heart disease) and cerebrovascular (stroke) complications of diabetes killed 193,000 Americans in 1996, the first year accurate data for diabetic mortality were calculated. A summary of the particulars is presented in Table 2.1.

Vascular complications of diabetes kill ten times as many people in the U.S. each year as do AIDS and breast cancer combined; ironically, Federal funding for diabetes research historically has been a fraction of that spent on these other serious conditions. The *American Diabetes Association* estimates that **diabetes costs the U.S. economy approximately $100 billion annually** due to direct medical expenses as well as indirect expenses related to lost productivity from hospitalization and disabling complications. This means that diabetes costs more than $9,000 per diagnosed case per year, or $285 per U.S. citizen per year.

Many experts believe that diabetes research is seriously under funded, especially when considering the numbers of people affected and the economic costs involved. The "Diabetes Research Working Group" (DRWG), a blue ribbon panel of diabetes researchers, epidemiologists and doctors appointed by the Secretary of Health and Human Services during the Clinton Administration, recommended federal funding of dia-

Table 2.1
The Epidemiology of Diabetes and Its Complications (all figures are approximate)

Total # of Americans with Diagnosed Diabetes   12.5 million   Total # with Type 1   1.5 million
Total # of Americans with Undiagnosed Diabetes 5 million   Total # with Type 2   16 million
Total # of Americans with Diabetes   17.5 million   17.5 million

Diabetes as a Cause of:	Annual Incidence (in US):	Rank:
Renal Failure	100,000	1st
Non-traumatic Amputation	80,000+	1st
	32,000 toes	1st
	12,000 feet	1st
	36,000 legs	1st
New Blindness*	22,000	1st
in persons < 74 years of age		(3rd leading cause of new blindness overall)
Death	69,000—300,000 (193,000)**	6th

*"Blindness" means "legal blindness," defined as best-corrected vision (i.e. with glasses or contact lenses) of less than 20/200 in the better seeing eye or less than 20 degrees of visual field (peripheral vision). Legally blind persons may have at least some useful vision. Diabetes accounts for roughly 22,000 cases of new legal blindness annually, with 8,000 of those being totally blinded (i.e. no useful vision).

** Studies show a range of mortality from diabetes, primarily because some use coroner reports listing diabetes as the "sole cause" of death (the 69,000 number), while other studies incorporate diabetes as either sole cause or a "contributing cause" of death (the 193,000 number is from CDC, Centers for Disease Control, statistics for 1996), while still others incorporate both, as well as a predicted rate of under-reporting (the 300,000 number). I will use the CDC number, 193,000 for my discussion.

betes research at a level of $1.3 billion in 2002 to prevent complications from and find a cure for diabetes. The current National Institutes of Health (NIH) budget has earmarked $770 million in fiscal 2002 for diabetes research, meaning that current research is under funded by nearly 41% compared with expert recommendations. Many members of the DRWG believe that finding a cure for diabetes is mostly a matter of finding enough money to fund already proposed research programs.

The Myth of Type 2 Benevolence

As Table 2.1 illustrates, the majority of diabetics are Type 2. What may surprise some readers is the fact that **the majority of diabetes complications are also found in Type 2 diabetics**.

There is a common perception among the general population, and Type 2 diabetics in particular, that Type 2 diabetes is less likely to cause complications than is Type 1 diabetes and, as such, is the "better kind" of diabetes to have (less worrisome, less dangerous etc.) In fact, *Type 1 diabetics* **are** *more prone to suffer many complications of diabetes, based on percentages, than are Type 2 diabetics*. This is especially true of the so-called "microvascular," or small blood vessel, complications like kidney disease and retinopathy (more on this later).

However, **the much larger number of Type 2 patients overall translates into many more Type 2 diabetics suffering complications than do Type 1 patients.** In addition, many Type 2 patients have risk factors, above and beyond those found in Type 1 patients, which increase the odds of suffering "macrovascular," or large blood vessel, complications such as heart disease (the main reason why diabetes is the sixth leading cause of death in the US). In fact, **Type 2 diabetics are two to four times more likely to die of heart disease**

compared with non-diabetics, and 22% more likely than Type 1 diabetics. The most serious complication of any medical condition is death. A serious argument can be made, therefore, that Type 2 diabetes is more worrisome than Type 1 diabetes, based upon the incidence of cardiovascular mortality alone.

The biological and chemical processes by which diabetes causes complications (known as the *pathophysiology*) are, in many ways, identical for all diabetics, both Type 1 and Type 2. In the absence of good diabetes control, the risk of complications for both groups is very high. Unfortunately, the myth of Type 2 benevolence fosters a false sense of security in many patients and their health care providers. There is no type of diabetes that is harmless. **Diabetes of any type is a serious medical condition, as Table 2.2 clearly demonstrates.**

Table 2.2
Diabetes Complications (US)
According to Type of Diabetes
(all figures are approximate)

Annual Incidence of:	Type 1	Type 2
Renal Failure	26,000	74,000
Non-traumatic amputations	24,500	55,500
New Blindness	10,000	12,000
Death	10,000	183,000
Total Complications	**70,500**	**313,500**
Total Complications as a percentage of diabetes Type	7.05%	1.97%* (2.63%)
Death Rate as a percentage of diabetes type	1%	1.22%

*This percentage is based upon the total number of Type 2 diabetics, both diagnosed and undiagnosed (17 million according to American Diabetes Association estimates). The percentage increases to 2.63 % if we use complications as a percentage of diagnosed Type 2 patients.

Key Points

1. More than seventeen million Americans have diabetes; Five million have not yet been diagnosed.

2. Diabetes is the leading cause of new blindness in People under 70, kidney failure and non-traumatic amputation. Diabetes is the sixth leading cause of death in the US.

3. Diabetes complications cost the US economy $100 billion annually.

4. Most complications of diabetes occur in Type 2 patients. Type 2 diabetes is not benevolent.

5. Both Type 1 and Type 2 diabetes are serious medical conditions.

Chapter Three:

Definitions and Pathophysiology Made Easy

This chapter will establish some fundamental definitions of diabetes and its subtypes, and explore the "pathophysiology," the chemical and biological mechanisms (physiology), by which diabetes causes damage to body tissues (pathology).

Diabetes is an endocrine disorder characterized by either a deficiency of endogenous insulin, a loss of cellular response to insulin, or both, resulting in a state of chronic hyperglycemia. This is a textbook definition of diabetes, but what does it really mean? Let's break it down.

Endocrine refers to *glands* in general but, more specifically, to glands that secrete chemical messengers, called "hormones," *directly into the blood stream* (as opposed to, for instance, glands that secrete substances directly to the surface of your skin, like sweat glands, or into your tears, like the eye's lacrimal gland — these glands are often called "exocrine" glands because they secrete outside of (exo-) the blood stream rather than into (endo-) the blood stream). Examples of endocrine glands include the pituitary, the thyroid, and the pancreas. Because these glands secrete directly into the circulatory system, their *effects are found throughout the body*, wherever blood flows. Conversely, a deficiency in any one of these secretions, whether it is growth hormone, thyroid hormone, insulin or any other endocrine substance, results in *body-wide* abnormalities called "endocrine disorders" or "endocrine diseases." Diabetes is an endocrine disorder involving the hormone insulin, normally secreted by the pancreas.

Endogenous means substances (in this case, the hormone insulin) naturally manufactured and secreted by the individual's *own body*. This is to be contrasted with "exogenous" insulin that is derived from external sources (including beef, pork and synthetic human insulin). Many diabetics are unable to produce enough (or any) of their own insulin, so they are said to have an "endogenous insulin deficiency." This is true of all Type 1 diabetics, and some Type 2 diabetics.

Figure 3.1

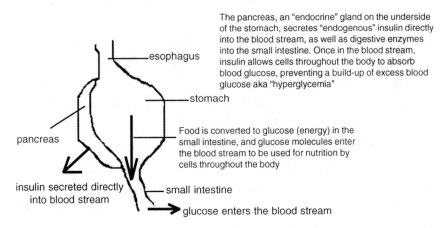

The pancreas, an "endocrine" gland on the underside of the stomach, secretes "endogenous" insulin directly into the blood stream, as well as digestive enzymes into the small intestine. Once in the blood stream, insulin allows cells throughout the body to absorb blood glucose, preventing a build-up of excess blood glucose aka "hyperglycemia"

esophagus

stomach

pancreas

Food is converted to glucose (energy) in the small intestine, and glucose molecules enter the blood stream to be used for nutrition by cells throughout the body

insulin secreted directly into blood stream

small intestine

glucose enters the blood stream

Normal Insulin Metabolism

What does "**a loss of cellular response to insulin**" mean? To understand this phrase, it is helpful to understand the basic role of cells and the role of insulin in normal physiology. All living tissue is comprised of cells, individual biological units that carry out specific functions and each of which contains genetic information within a nucleus at its center. Cells are often "differentiated," meaning that groups of particular kinds of cells perform very specialized and/or unique tasks and may be physically concentrated within a particular body organ. Examples include cardiac (heart muscle) cells whose function is to continuously pump blood, hepatic (liver) cells which remove toxic substances from the blood, and pancreatic cells, some of which specialize in producing insulin (these specialized pancreatic cells are known as the *Islets of Langerhans* or, more simply, *islet cells*.)

All cells within the body require a source of energy, which, generally speaking, comes from the foods we eat. Once in the digestive tract, sugar molecules, also known as glucose, are extracted from food and enter the blood stream after absorption by the small intestine. A more or less constant level of blood glucose continuously circulates throughout the body in order to provide the body's billions of cells with a source of readily available energy.

To use blood sugar for energy, however, requires that cells bring glucose "inside" of them for nourishment (analogous to the way we must consume food to derive nourishment, we can't just look at or smell it!) Bringing glucose "inside" means that cell membranes (the outer wall of cells, so to speak) must become permeable to blood glucose, a process which must be tightly regulated by the body, as either too much or too little glucose on the inside (called *intracellular glucose*) can cause cellular damage or cellular death. The "door" leading to the inside of each cell must be controlled so that it is not too wide open and not too narrow to allow the proper amount of glucose inside. This door, to continue the analogy, is regulated by insulin, which acts like a "key" to unlock the cell membrane to the passage of blood glucose. The "lock" on the surface of the cell membrane consists of a particular region, with a unique three-dimensional structure, that allows insulin molecules to attach; this region is known as the *insulin recep-*

tor site, and is specifically configured to accept insulin molecules only, much the same way a specific key is designed to fit a specific lock, and that lock only (figure 3.2).

Figure 3.2
Insulin Receptor Site on a Cell

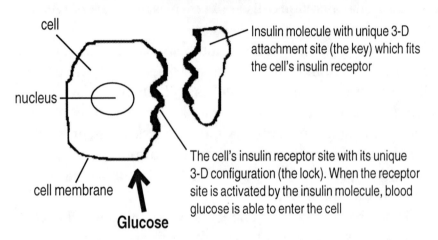

cell

Insulin molecule with unique 3-D attachment site (the key) which fits the cell's insulin receptor

nucleus

The cell's insulin receptor site with its unique 3-D configuration (the lock). When the receptor site is activated by the insulin molecule, blood glucose is able to enter the cell

cell membrane

Glucose

Insulin Resistance and Hyperinsulinemia

In some Type 2 diabetics, insulin receptor sites become unresponsive to insulin, a condition known as **"insulin resistance."** Insulin (the key) will no longer bind, or have difficulty binding, to the receptor site (the lock), like a car key that doesn't quite fit an old or defective door lock anymore. Without insulin, the cell membrane (the door) remains impermeable (closed) to blood glucose, and the cell is unable to receive adequate glucose to perform its functions. Glucose remains in the bloodstream, where it builds up to excessive amounts, a condition known as **"hyperglycemia."** Eventually, the body produces (if it is able) more insulin in an attempt to overcome poorly responsive cellular insulin receptors (in essence, to force the lock open), and blood sugar levels begin to normalize. This entire process may be summed up as a "loss of cellular response to insulin," and plays an important role in many Type 2 diabetics.

To further complicate the situation, the liver of many Type 2 patients begins to secrete the hormone glycogen, which causes the liver to release glucose and raises blood sugar levels even higher. When cells are unable to receive adequate nourishment (glucose) due to a loss of cellular response to insulin, the pancreas releases glucagon, a hormone that stimulates the liver to produce glycogen, and a vicious cycle is created of inadequate intracellular glucose, elevated blood sugar (hyperglycemia) due to both a loss of cellular insulin response and further glucose release by the liver, and elevated endogenous insulin production (a condition known as "*hyperinsulinemia*"). Figure 3.3 illustrates this vicious cycle.

Figure 3.3
Vicious Cycle of Insulin Resistance, Chronic Hyperglycemia & Hyperinsulinemia

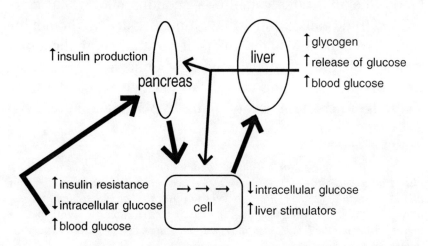

Type 1 and Type 2 Diabetes

Now that we have basic understanding of what diabetes is, we are in a much better position to consider the definitions of Type 1 and Type 2 diabetes, and the complications caused by each. **In Type 1 diabetes, there is no endogenous insulin production, due to either failure of, or destruction of, the pancreatic islet cells**. Most cases of type 1 diabetes are due to *autoimmunity*; that is, the body's own immune system treats the pancreatic islet cells as a foreign substance and destroys them. Without insulin, blood glucose is unable to get inside of cells, and a state of chronic hyperglycemia results, which may then easily spiral out of control to cause severely acute hyperglycemia. This is why all Type 1 diabetics must receive "exogenous insulin" (typically in the form of injections or via catheter from a mechanical insulin pump), and are said to be "insulin dependant."*

Without exogenous insulin, Type 1 patients are subject to tremendous elevations in blood sugar levels in a relatively short period of time (hours to days). Left untreated, this condition leads to the production of "ketones," a very dangerous by-product of abnormal metabolism that lowers the pH of the blood (making it more acidic — a condition known as *keto-acidosis*) and causes coma and, ultimately, death. Though life saving, treatment with insulin itself can cause complications, the most obvious of which is hypoglycemia, low blood sugar, which is incapacitating and, if left unchecked, can be fatal. **Aside from the dangers of acute hyperglycemia and hy-**

---

* *It should be mentioned, in fact emphasized, that cellular glucose metabolism is also regulated by physical activity. Exercise, even in the total absence of insulin, allows most (but not all) cell membranes to absorb blood glucose and thereby lowers blood sugar. When insulin is present, exercise makes it more effective, thereby lowering the body's insulin requirement. Exercise is, indeed, a very important aspect of good blood sugar control.*

poglycemia, most complications from Type 1 diabetes occur as a result of *chronic* hyperglycemia.

Type 2 diabetics, by contrast, have at least *some* endogenous insulin production, and very often suffer a loss of
cellular response to insulin, or "insulin resistance." A *relative* loss of insulin production and/or insulin resistance is the
hallmark of Type 2 diabetes. So there are really three subcategories of Type 2 diabetes: (1) A decrease in the normal production of insulin, but normal cellular response to insulin, (2) A decrease in the normal production of insulin combined with a loss of cellular response to insulin, or (3) Normal insulin production with a loss of cellular response to insulin. It is believed that most Type 2 diabetics fall under
subcategory 2 — a decrease of normal insulin production
in tandem with insulin resistance.

Note that in two of these subcategories, there is a decrease
in normal insulin production, and in another two, a loss of
cellular response to insulin — both problems which can occur for a variety of different reasons, but are often related
to obesity. With increased body weight there is an increased
demand on the pancreas to produce insulin for regulating intracellular glucose (since there is a larger amount of body tissue and increased number of cells.) This can lead to a relative
insulin deficiency because the pancreas is unable to "keep up"
with the excessive demand, or because islet cells that *can* meet
the increased demand *initially* eventually lose capacity (i.e. burn
out, run out of gas, as it were.) Obesity is thought to increase
insulin resistance because of changes in metabolism which alter the unique and finicky three-dimensional structure of cellular insulin receptors (changes which "strip the lock" so that the
"key," insulin, no longer fits very well.) When coupled with
relative insulin deficiency, this insulin resistance becomes even
more problematic.

Because these patients are still capable of making their own
insulin, medical therapy has often aimed at stimulating the

pancreas to produce more insulin, using oral medications. The problem is a relative under-production of insulin, not a total loss of production, as in Type 1 patients. Other therapies are directed at reducing insulin resistance, decreasing hepatic (liver) production of glucose, receiving additional exogenous insulin (i.e. injections), and slowing down the absorption of glucose via the small intestine. Very often, therapy includes a combination of these treatments, each of which has its particular advantages and disadvantages. Left untreated, chronic hyperglycemia develops but usually acute hyperglycemia and profound keto-acidosis do not (as in untreated Type 1 patients). **As mentioned earlier, elevated levels of insulin in the blood stream are commonly found in many of these patients** (as the body compensates for increased cellular mass — as occurs with obesity, or as the body tries to force open the lock on cellular insulin receptors by producing more insulin, in effect, by making more keys to fit the lock — as occurs with insulin resistance, or for both of these reasons.) What often begins as a disease at least partially caused by a *lack* of insulin production, paradoxically can become a disease of *excessive* insulin production. **Complications from Type 2 diabetes arise from chronic hyperglycemia (as in Type 1) and insulin resistance/hyperinsulinemia (a feature more typical of Type 2 diabetes.)**

The Effects of Chronic Hyperglycemia and Insulin Resistance

So why, it seems reasonable to ask, is **hyperglycemia** bad for the body? Also, why is **insulin resistance/ hyperinsulinemia (excess insulin in the blood stream)** a bad thing? As we have seen, acute hyperglycemia can lead to keto-acidosis and coma, obviously bad things. But why is chronic hyperglycemia such a bad thing? **Over time, hyperglycemia**

**causes many diabetes complications by damaging the small-
est, most fragile blood vessels of the body. Such blood vessels are found in large numbers in the long nerves of the
legs and feet, the kidneys, and the eyes.** High levels of blood
glucose disrupt the integrity (strength) of these smallest blood
vessels, allowing blood and some of its components (primarily serum, the watery part of blood) to leak out of them into
the surrounding tissue, causing the release of inflammatory
chemical messengers which further damage those tissues, and
depriving them of an adequate blood supply via normal circulation. **Because the smallest blood vessels are damaged,
this cascade of events is referred to as "micro-vascular disease"** (figure 3.4)

Figure 3.4
Micro-Vascular Damage
Caused by Chronic Hyperglycemia

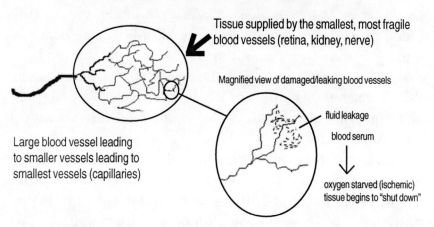

Tissue supplied by the smallest, most fragile blood vessels (retina, kidney, nerve)

Magnified view of damaged/leaking blood vessels

Large blood vessel leading to smaller vessels leading to smallest vessels (capillaries)

fluid leakage

blood serum

oxygen starved (ischemic) tissue begins to "shut down"

When tissue (and the cells it contains) receives inadequate
circulation, a condition called "ischemia" (pronounced ih-
skeem-ee-ah), cells begin to die because they are receiving
inadequate nourishment (glucose) and oxygen from the blood
stream. The death of individual cells, in turn, releases more

inflammatory chemical messengers and another vicious cycle begins. Even when the hyperglycemia is treated, cellular damage continues until the body is able to compensate for the ischemia by growing new blood vessels and/or "shutting down" ischemic tissues. By way of extension, this is exactly what happens in "ischemic heart disease" (i.e. heart attack, or "myocardial infarction"). When heart muscle receives inadequate blood supply (ischemia), typically due to clogged blood vessels within the heart, the affected part of the heart stops functioning (shuts down) and, in addition, the heart tries to develop new blood vessels in an attempt to redirect circulation around the diseased area. Ischemic heart disease is an example of a "macro-vascular" (large blood vessel) compromise to blood circulation.

In the long nerves of the legs and feet, "shutting down" means that nerves no longer function properly, resulting in loss of sensation ("hypoesthesia") or abnormal sensation (feeling of pins and needles or tingling, called "paresthesia.") In the kidneys, it means that cells are no longer able to filter blood properly and maintain proper fluid balance; it means kidney dysfunction and, ultimately, kidney failure requiring dialysis or transplantation. In the eyes it means, among many things, that retinal tissue dies, causing permanent "blind spots" and triggering the growth of abnormal blood vessels that can lead to blindness.

It is important to note that **chronic hyperglycemia plays an important role in causing the micro-vascular (small blood vessel) complications of both Type 1 and Type 2 diabetes.** The more elevated blood glucose levels are on a chronic basis, and the longer the body has had to sustain the insults of hyperglycemia, the higher the odds of suffering these micro-vascular complications. **This is a general rule of diabetes and its complications; the longer you've had it, and the farther your blood sugars stray from normal levels, the higher the risk.** In the eyes, for instance, the prevalence (overall occurrence) of retinopathy after ten years is about 60%, but after 20 years is over 90%. Moreover, each 10% elevation in average blood sugar level increases the risk of retinopathy by as much as 65% (more on the specifics of diabetic eye disease, including diabetic retinopathy, in Section II.)

What about insulin resistance and hyperinsulinemia? (defined as "elevated levels of freely circulating insulin.") Much investigation has centered on the reasons why diabetic patients, particularly Type 2 patients, experience a much higher rate of macro-vascular (both cardiovascular and cerebrovascular) diseases than do non-diabetics of the same age (again, we're talking about heart disease and stroke, the first and third leading killers of *all* Americans.) **Research suggests that excess insulin levels in the blood stream raise blood pressure and impair the *normal* breakdown of blood clots, both of which increase the risk of macrovascular disease by enhancing the formation of "atheromas," accumulations of fatty deposits within the walls of blood vessels** which predispose those vessels to occlusion (blockage) and production of fatty emboli (clots that break free and travel within the circulatory system to lodge at another location.) Atheromas typically form in the large arteries of the heart, the neck, and the legs (occlusions of the latter cause what is called "peripheral vascular disease.")

In addition, patients with insulin resistance tend to have higher levels of both triglycerides (blood fats) and LDL cholesterol (the "bad," plaque forming kind of cholesterol) that further predispose them to macro-vascular disease. Perhaps more importantly, *LDL cholesterol in many Type 2 diabetics is abnormal, consisting of smaller, denser particles than those found in non-diabetics, a feature that further promotes formation of atheromas*.

When "atheromatous plaques" occlude coronary arteries, for instance, the heart muscle they nourish becomes compromised and may die (a heart attack has occurred). When emboli break off an atheroma within the carotid artery, which supplies circulation to the head, they can travel to and become lodged within the smaller blood vessels of the brain, causing ischemia and death to that part of the brain (a "cerebrovascular accident," AKA a stroke has occurred.) **This entire process is accelerated in diabetics as a result of insulin resistance, abnormal blood lipid profile and hyperinsulinemia**. This is not to say that hyperinsulinemia and lipid abnormalities with an increased risk of macro-vascular disease don't occur in Type 1 patients (for example, patients taking unusually high dosages of injected insulin to cover high caloric intake, or Type 1 patients with abnormal blood lipid profiles), only that it is much more common in Type 2 patients, and especially in those with insulin resistance (figure 3.5)

Figure 3.5
Macro-Vascular Damage Resulting From Abnormal Blood Lipids and Hyperinsulinemia

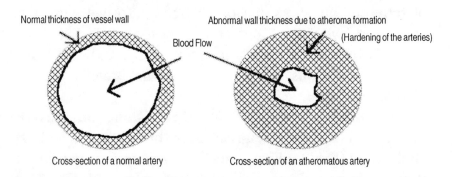

Normal thickness of vessel wall   Abnormal wall thickness due to atheroma formation

Blood Flow   (Hardening of the arteries)

Cross-section of a normal artery   Cross-section of an atheromatous artery

Abnormal blood lipid profile (high triglycerides + high/abnormal LDL cholesterol) combined with excessive insulin (hyperinsulinemia) accelerates atheroma formation AKA "atherosclerosis," resulting in reduced blood flow through large vessels (e.g. in the heart) and greatly increasing macro-vascular disease (i.e. heart disease, stroke, and blood clots)

To review, hyperinsulinemia occurs in some Type 2 patients as the pancreas increases insulin production in an attempt to compensate for insulin resistance (the loss of cellular response to insulin) and the chronic hyperglycemia that ensues. Research has shown that hyperinsulinemia and insulin resistance are each *independent* risk factors for macrovascular disease, and that their combined detrimental effect is greater than either one by itself. **This group of factors - insulin resistance, hyperglycemia and hyperinsulinemia, coupled with an abnormal blood lipid profile and increased risk of macro-vascular disease (heart disease, stroke and peripheral vascular disease), is often referred to as "Syndrome X."**

Medications that significantly increase the production of endogenous insulin beyond normal levels, we might expect, would similarly increase the likelihood of diabetic macrovascular complications, as would exogenous insulin (insulin injections), *if* the person in question has a normally functioning pancreas (and therefore is not truly insulin deficient.) In other words, hyperinsulinemia only occurs when insulin levels are above and beyond those produced by a normally functioning pancreas.

The role of hyperinsulinemia in promoting cardiovascular disease is somewhat controversial, however, as some major studies (including the landmark "United Kingdom Prospective Diabetes Study") *have not* revealed an increased risk amongst Type 2 patients receiving either insulin or drug therapy that increases endogenous production of insulin. **In fact, there is a wide range of "normal" insulin levels within the non-diabetic population, and some studies are showing a link between higher levels of circulating insulin in *non-diabetics* and an increased risk of heart disease.** Indeed, there is mounting evidence that the production and regulation of insulin may play a large role in the epidemic of macrovascular diseases seen in the United States and the entire Western World. Hyperinsulinemia seen in diabetes may be just the tip of the iceberg.

Of course, an abnormal blood lipid profile leads to atheroma formation and macro-vascular disease in many individuals (probably *most* individuals in the Western World), diabetics and non-diabetics alike. Control of these factors is often amenable to improved diet, exercise and medical (drug) intervention, as well as strict avoidance of smoking, but to the extent diabetics have a higher likelihood of developing this abnormal blood lipid profile compared to the general population, their risk will be higher as well.

Clinical Diagnosis of Diabetes

The clinical diagnosis of diabetes is predicated upon *hyperglycemia* (primarily), as demonstrated by laboratory measurement of *Fasting Plasma Glucose* (FPG), *Random Plasma Glucose* (RPG) or *Oral Glucose Tolerance Test* (OGTT). FPG indicates how much glucose (sugar) is present in a specific amount of plasma (blood with the red blood cells removed by centrifuge) after the patient has fasted (has had no caloric intake for 8 hours), and is customarily measured as milligrams of glucose per deciliter of plasma (abbreviated mg/dl; a milligram is roughly 1/30,000th of an ounce; a deciliter is a little over 3 fluid ounces). RPG is the same test without fasting or regard for food consumption. The OGTT requires the patient to consume a specific amount of glucose (essentially sugar water), after fasting, with measurement of plasma glucose 2 hours later (this test has fallen out of favor with many physicians.)

As an interesting aside, home blood glucose meters measure *whole blood glucose* (because the red blood cells are still present), the values of which are lower than plasma glucose by about 15% (some glucose meters are calibrated to convert whole blood glucose measurements into plasma glucose readings, allowing patients to compare home readings more accurately with laboratory readings.)

The "classic" symptoms of diabetes (due strictly to hyper-glycemia) are *polyuria* (frequent and excessive urination), *polydipsia* (excessive thirst), and *weight loss*. When blood glucose levels rise significantly, excess glucose is spilled (leeches out) into urine being processed by the kidneys, which draws more fluid from the blood stream and the body's cells. This leads to a larger volume of urine and dehydration, causing thirst. Weight loss occurs as urine output increases and because the body's cells are unable to receive adequate nourishment. Other symptoms frequently experienced are fluctuating vision, headache, nausea, irritability and slow healing.

The required standard for a clinical diagnosis of diabetes is one of the following:

1. **FPG greater than 126 mg/dl on two or more occasions**
2. **RPG greater than 200 mg/dl when accompanied by symptoms of polyuria, polydipsia, and/or unexplained weight loss**
3. **OGTT readings above 200 mg/dl at two hours**

If one (or more) of these criteria is met, the person in question has diabetes. Period. Values near but below these mean an individual has "impaired glucose tolerance," or "pre-diabetes" (a new classification meaning that patients have FPG or RPG values above normal, but not abnormal enough to be diagnosed with diabetes. The *American Diabetes Association* estimates that as many as 16 million Americans have "pre-diabetes.") In non-diabetics, FPG is typically 65-90 mg/dl, RPG is 70-110 mg/dl and OGTT is under 160 mg/dl. These values are based upon clinical and laboratory experience with millions of patients, though there have been some small changes made over the years to accommodate that experience and the recommendations of diabetes experts.

Hemoglobin A-1-c

This test measures the overall quality of a patient's blood sugar control over an 8 to 12 week period of time, and is considered to be **the single most important laboratory test for all diabetic patients.** The test goes by several different names: glycosylated hemoglobin, glycated hemoglobin, glycohemoglobin, and hemoglobin A-1-c (abbreviated HbA1c). **This test averages the minute-by-minute changes in a person's blood sugar levels over two to three months, and *correlates very highly with the risk of diabetes complications.*** It's essentially the same as poking your finger and measuring your home blood glucose levels *every minute of every day* for at least two solid months, and then averaging all (86,400) of those readings. Obviously, this gives a much better picture of overall blood sugar control than one, or two, or four, or even ten individual blood glucose measurements per day! Home blood glucose testing is *no* substitute for having this test regularly.

Hemoglobin is the part of red blood cells responsible for carrying oxygen to all parts of the body. In addition to carrying oxygen, glucose in the bloodstream also becomes attached (bound) to hemoglobin molecules. HbA1c testing works by measuring the amount of blood glucose that is bound to hemoglobin molecules (the "A1c" part of hemoglobin molecules) on the red blood cells circulating throughout our bodies. Because individual red blood cells normally last only 8 to 12 weeks, the amount of glucose bound to old red blood cells (expressed as a percentage) shows the average blood glucose level over that period of time.

Normal HbA1c values are 4-6% (equivalent to a blood glucose average of 60-120 mg/dl). An easy way to figure out what percentage equals what blood glucose level is to remember that an HbA1c of 6% equals a blood glucose average of 120 mg/dl, and that every 1% (1 unit) change in HbA1c correlates with a 30 mg/dl change in average blood glucose (so a 7% equals 150, a 5% equals 90, a 9.5% equals 225 mg/dl, and so on.) Most diabetes doctors recommend that patients strive to keep their HbA1c values under 7.5% (a 165 mg/dl average), and the *American Diabetes Association* recommends they be kept at 7.0% or less (a 150 mg/dl average), provided there are no medical reasons (for example, severe heart disease) to avoid this.

What Really Causes Diabetes?

The title of this chapter makes an implied promise that the material presented will be easy to understand, and I apologize to the reader if that promise has not been totally fulfilled. The pathophysiology of diabetes is, in fact, a complicated subject, with many twists and turns that some readers will have difficulty following. **Do not be discouraged**. Doctors and other scientists get confused by these convolutions as well. Truth be told, this chapter has barely delved into the many intricacies of diabetes and the various ways in which the body responds to it. Hopefully, though, it has laid a strong foundation for understanding the **true fundamentals** of diabetes, the fundamentals as they are understood by clinical and research diabetes experts, enabling you to reach a fuller understanding of diabetes, its classifications, the ways in which it causes complications, and the rationale underlying its various treatments.

This entire chapter, of course, begs the question **"What really causes diabetes?"** In some sense, we have answered that question by understanding, *physiologically*, what goes

wrong inside the bodies of diabetic persons. We can identify
the exact chemical and biological processes that "cause" diabetes. We know, for instance, that Type 1 patients have circulating antibodies against the pancreatic "beta cells" (the particular islet cells which produce insulin), demonstrating the
autoimmune nature of this condition. We know much about
the genetic influences associated with Type 2 diabetes and
will, no doubt, learn much more in the future.

These sorts of explanations are not entirely satisfactory,
however, because they don't explain why these processes
occur in some individuals and not in others. Even if we
establish a genetic or hereditary basis for diabetes, which
scientific investigation surely has, we are still left to pon-
der why those genes are activated in one family member
and not another. Even if we demonstrate environmental factors that contribute to the development of diabetes, which,
again, science certainly has, we can point to people with
those same environmental risk factors who don't develop
diabetes. Even a combination explanation, attributing diabetes to both heredity and environment, doesn't always
account for individual cases of diabetes.

Establishing causality can be murky and confusing, not
just because there may be many different causes that interact
in complex and confusing ways, but because there are many
different levels of explanation for any "event," some of which
are "scientific," some of which are "religious" and/or "spiri-
tual," and many of which are both or neither. Every explanation or cause raises a thousand new questions, and may leave
us wondering "Why" or "What Caused *That* Cause?" As it
turns out, science is not able to explain to each person's satis-
faction the ultimate causes of all things, even those that are
expressly within the purview of scientific knowledge. This is
the nature of the world and the language we humans use to
describe and explain it. When someone asks about the cause
of diabetes, she or he is usually asking "Why did I get diabe-

tes?" or "Why does somebody I love have diabetes?" What constitutes a satisfactory answer will depend, ultimately, on what kinds of explanations we are looking for.

Key Points

1. Diabetes is a disease involving insulin metabolism that results in hyperglycemia (high blood sugar).

2. Type 1 diabetes is caused by the body's inability to produce any of its own insulin.

3. Type 2 diabetes is caused by either a relative lack of insulin production, a loss of the body's ability to use insulin properly, or both.

4. Chronic hyperglycemia causes damage to the smallest blood vessels found in the nerves, kidneys and eyes. This is true of both Type 1 and Type 2 diabetes.

5. Many Type 2 diabetics have an excess of freely circulating insulin (hyperinsulinemia) and abnormal blood lipid profiles, the combination of which appears to significantly increase the risk of heart disease and stroke.

6. The risk of diabetes complications increases the longer a person has had diabetes, and the higher her average blood sugar levels are over time.

7. The cause of diabetes, from a scientific perspective, is a combination of genetic and environmental factors that remain to be fully explained.

Chapter Four:

The Major Diabetes Studies

N ow that we have a solid foundation for understanding the pathophysiology of diabetes and its complications, we will consider what scientific research has taught us about how to best prevent those complications or, at least, to mini- mize them. As I was growing up with diabetes, I was often told to keep my sugar levels (initially, urine glucose levels, later, blood glucose levels) as close to normal as possible, in hope of preventing long-term complications. However, no one was ever able to offer solid evidence that doing so made any real difference; certainly, no one was able to quantify that difference. I remember well my human physiology profes- sor, during my freshman year in college, saying that he thought blood sugar control made little difference to the long-term prospects of diabetic patients, as complications were "inevi- table." I am happy to report that, now, there *is* excellent sci- entific evidence, and that my (Ivy League) physiology pro- fessor was "flat out wrong."

There are two ground breaking, landmark studies that have investigated the complications of diabetes, over time and in a large number of patients, as a function of blood sugar con- trol. One of them, the DCCT, focused only on Type 1 diabe- tes while the other, the UKPDS, focused exclusively on Type 2 diabetes. The results of these studies are constantly referred to in medical literature, and some educational materials pri- marily aimed at patients and their families. Importantly, much of the rationale behind good diabetes management and state-of-the-art medical care is derived from these studies, so it will be useful to have some familiarity with them.

The Diabetes Control and Complication Trial (DCCT)

The "Diabetes Control and Complication Trial" was conducted in the United States and Canada from 1983-1993, and involved 1,441 Type 1 diabetics. The primary aim of the study was to answer a critical question regarding the effectiveness of tight blood sugar control on the likelihood of developing complications from Type 1 diabetes. **Specifically, the DCCT compared the rate of complications and the worsening of complications between a group of patients receiving "intensive treatment" and another receiving "conventional treatment" for Type 1 diabetes.** To qualify for the study, patients had to have Type 1 diabetes for between 1.5 and 15 years, be over the age of 13 (average age was 27), and have suffered no or minimal complications due to diabetes (e.g. patients with a minimal degree of diabetic retinopathy were accepted into the study, but patients with advanced retinopathy were excluded.)

After receiving a one-month educational program on diabetes management, patients were divided randomly into two groups and then followed over the course of the study for the development of complications. Due to the drop out of some study participants (a feature of virtually all large scale studies), complication rates were followed over a period of time ranging from five to nine years. All volunteer patients were receiving standard treatment prior to enrollment in the study, meaning one or two insulin injections daily.

The first group underwent a regimen of "intensive management," defined by the study as: three or more insulin injections daily *or* the use of an insulin pump, with insulin dosages adjusted according to a sliding scale of blood sugar readings (i.e. the higher the reading, the larger the dose of insulin taken), dietary intake and exercise; four or more home blood glucose measurements daily; monthly evaluations by a team of diabetes specialists including a medical doctor specializing in diabetes, diabetes nurse educator, dietician and behavioral therapist; frequent phone consultations with these same specialists, who were available on a 24 hour basis.

The second group of patients received "conventional therapy," consisting of one or two daily insulin injections, daily self-monitoring of blood glucose or urine glucose, physician consultations every three months, and intensive treatment *only* in female patients becoming pregnant during the course of the study (the risk of diabetes complications worsening during pregnancy, and risk of fetal injury, were well known at the study's inception.)

At the study conclusion in 1993, the mean (average) glycosylated hemoglobin (HbA1c) level of the intensively managed group over the period of the study was 7.2% (equivalent to an average blood plasma glucose level of 156mg/dl), while the mean level of the conventionally treated group was 9% (equivalent to an average blood plasma glucose level of 210 mg/dl.) Normal HbA1c values (in non-diabetic individuals) range from 4-6% (average blood plasma glucose level of 60-120mg/dl.)

As compared to the conventional treatment group, the intensive treatment group had a 76% reduced risk of developing diabetic retinopathy and a 54% reduced risk of worsening retinopathy (in those who had early stages of retinopathy at the beginning of the study), a 50% reduced risk of developing and worsening diabetic nephropathy (kidney disease), and a 60% reduced risk of developing diabetic neuropathy (nerve disease). There was no evidence that intensive treatment reduced the risk of worsening neuropathy in patients with preexisting diabetic

A. Paul Chous

nerve disease. Though few cases of cardiovascular disease occurred in the young study population, too few to demonstrate a statistically significant (*or insignificant*) reduction in risk, **intensive treatment did lower the risk of developing high cholesterol by 22%**. To the extent that high cholesterol is a contributor to heart disease, we can infer that this reduction in risk would eventually translate into a reduction of cardiovascular disease (though the DCCT does *not* prove this.)

Patients receiving intensive treatment also experienced a three times (300%) greater risk of developing severe episodes of hypoglycemia (low blood sugar — "severe" defined as requiring the assistance of another person), and a 50% greater risk of gaining enough weight to be considered "overweight." In reporting their findings, DCCT researchers estimate that intensive management doubles the cost of managing diabetes due to increased medical visits and blood glucose testing supplies, but that such costs will be offset by a reduction in medical expenses as a result of fewer long-term diabetes complications as well as improved quality of life for people with diabetes. Table 4.1 summarizes the essential results of the Diabetes Control and Complications Trial.

Table 4.1
Results of the DCCT

Complication	Reduction in Risk for Intensive vs. Conventional Treatment
Diabetic Retinopathy	76%
Diabetic Nephropathy	50%
Diabetic Neuropathy	60%
Development of High Cholesterol	22%
Severe Hypoglycemic Episodes	-300% (3x *more* likely to occur)

A follow-up study to the DCCT, **the EDIC study** ("Epidemiology of Diabetes Interventions and Complications" study) tracked retinal and kidney complications of 1,375 DCCT participants for an additional four years, and showed that *the lower incidence of complications in the intensively treated group persisted during those four years, even though the HbA1c measurements for the two groups moved much closer together* (the intensively treated group's glycemic control worsened a bit, and the conventional group's control improved a bit.) This finding strongly suggests that improved glycemic control has a prolonged effect on the risk of developing microvascular diabetes complications (i.e. good blood sugar control has a *delayed* protective effect which extends into subsequent years.)

It is often stated that the DCCT **proved** that tight blood sugar control (as evidenced by HbA1c) reduces diabetes complications. This is not entirely accurate. The study compares intensive management with conventional management, and it certainly can be stated that the former was associated with a lower risk of certain diabetes complications as well as reduced HbA1c values, but not that reduced HbA1c *causes* fewer complications. The point may sound academic, but it is at least *conceivable* that other aspects of intensive management, for instance the team of diabetes experts working so closely with the patient, influenced complication rates in some fashion apart from reducing HbA1c values (the lead authors actually make this point in a paper published after the DCCT.) Furthermore, the DCCT did not study patients having advanced microvascular complications, those having had diabetes for more than 15 years, or (obviously) any Type 2 patients. The DCCT did show convincingly, though, that intensive management, with a goal of normalizing blood glucose levels as much as possible, delays the onset and slows the progression of long-term diabetic microvascular complications.

The United Kingdom Prospective
Diabetes Study (UKPDS)

Fortunately, the risk of diabetes complications for the majority of patients, Type 2 diabetics, was investigated by the "United Kingdom Prospective Diabetes Study" (UKPDS). Like the DCCT that preceded it, **the UKPDS evaluated the effectiveness of tight blood sugar control on reducing the risk of diabetes complications. In addition, this study addressed the impact of tight *blood pressure* control on complications, and produced some surprising results. Rigorous blood glucose and blood pressure control each were found to reduce significantly the risk of diabetic microvascular complications (retinopathy and nephropathy, and to a lesser degree, neuropathy), and tight blood pressure control was shown to significantly reduce the likelihood of cardiovascular disease and death in Type 2 diabetics with high blood pressure.**

The UKPDS studied more than 5000 newly diagnosed Type 2 diabetics from 1977 to 1997, dividing these patients into two groups: those receiving "intensive treatment" (defined as adherence to a diet in combination with insulin therapy and/or oral medications — either sulfonylureas or metformin — with a goal of achieving near normal blood glucose levels), and "conventional treatment" (defined as dietary and exercise control of blood sugar levels only — with a much more liberal, in other words, higher blood sugar target considered "acceptable"). During the study, many patient's blood sugar levels became too high to continue them with conventional treatment (diet and exercise only), so a fair number of participants were switched over to treatment with medication(s) and/or insulin; nonetheless, enough study participants remained in each group to demonstrate that **lower HbA1c levels (regardless of the methods used to achieve them) resulted in a 25% reduced risk of microvascular diabetes complications overall.**

Most of this benefit resulted from a decreased incidence of diabetic retinopathy severe enough to require laser treatment (more on this in Chapter 11.) The median HbA1c of the conventional treatment group was 7.9% (equivalent to a 177 mg/dl average) while that of the intensive treatment group was 7% (a 150 mg/dl average). **Each 1% drop in HbA1c (for example, from 9% to 8%, or from 8% to 7%) lowered the risk of death due to diabetes by 25%.** These decreases in risk were seen until HbA1c levels approached "normal" (defined as 6.2%, or an average blood glucose of 126 mg/dl).

As a separate part of the UKPDS, Type 2 diabetics with high blood pressure were divided in two additional groups: those treated intensively (with one or more medications) to achieve tight blood pressure control and those treated conventionally (with one or more medications) to achieve less tight control. The average blood pressure of the intensive group was 144/82, and that of the conventional group was 154/87. Even with such a small difference in average blood pressure readings, **the intensive treatment group had a 34% lowered risk of substantial worsening of diabetic retinopathy, *independent* of blood sugar control, a 49% reduced risk of significant loss of vision on the eye chart, a 44% lowered risk of stroke, and a 32% reduction in death caused by diabetes. Wow!** A 21% reduction in risk for heart attack was not statistically significant (meaning that given the number of patients studied, the lower incidence of heart attack may have been due purely to random chance), although it is encouraging. Table 4.2 summarizes some of the important results of the UKPDS.

Table 4.2
Results of the UKPDS

Complication	Reduction in Risk for Intensive vs. Conventional Glucose Control
Diabetic Retinopathy	25%
Diabetic Nephropathy	33%
Death Caused by Diabetes	25%
Severe Hypoglycemic Episodes	-200% (twice as likely to occur)

	Reduction in Risk for Intensive vs. Conventional Blood Pressure Control
Worsening Retinopathy	34%
Reduction in Vision	49%
Death Caused by Diabetes	32%
Stroke	44%

The UKPDS demonstrates that tight control of blood pressure and blood sugar are equally important in preventing microvascular diabetes complications, and that tight blood pressure control greatly reduces the risk of macrovascular diabetes complications. Moreover, intensive blood glucose control was not associated (as some other studies had shown) with an increased risk of cardiovascular disease, despite higher levels of circulating insulin in this group of patients. Significantly, obese Type 2 patients treated with metformin (Glucophage) experienced a much lower risk of cardiovascular disease compared to those treated with diet, sulfonylurea drugs or insulin. As with the DCCT, patients with more advanced eye, kidney, nerve and cardiovascular disease were not studied. Most (80%) of patients were unable to maintain acceptable blood glucose levels with diet and exercise alone, and there was a definite trend for blood glucose (HbA1c) levels to rise over time, leading to the conclusion that, for most Type 2 patients, good medical care will require multiple blood glucose medications over time.

Eye Studies

Two other very important clinical studies specifically pertaining to diabetic eye disease should be mentioned, and will be discussed again in Chapter 11: the **"Diabetic Retinopathy Study"** showed that laser treatment of severe (proliferative) diabetic retinopathy reduces the risk of "severe" vision loss (20/800 or worse on the eye chart, with glasses) by 50-75%; the **"Early Treatment of Diabetic Retinopathy Study"** showed that laser treatment of severe diabetic macular edema (another type of retinopathy) reduces the risk of less severe vision loss (defined as a 50% loss of vision on the eye chart — for example, worsening from 20/40 to 20/80 vision) by about 50%.

Key Points

1. **We now have excellent scientific evidence that the risk of complications from diabetes can be reduced significantly by better control of blood sugar, and using methods and medications that are currently available.**

2. **"Intensive" blood glucose control may not be good for all diabetics (The DCCT authors do not recommend it for patients under 13 years old, and the UKPDS authors do not recommend it for patients with serious heart disease), but it probably is good for most diabetics.**

3. **"Tight control" of even mild high blood pressure has been shown to greatly benefit Type 2 diabetics, and must be given high priority.**

Section Two:

Diabetic Eye Disease

Introduction:

Diabetic Eye Disease

In this section, we will consider in some detail the several different forms of diabetic eye disease, building upon the fundamentals discussed in previous chapters and stressing the steps every diabetic can and should take to reduce the risk of eye complications. Importantly, many of these risk reduction strategies will have the added benefit of reducing the risk of *all* diabetes complications, both microvascular (eyes, kidneys and nerves) and macrovascular (heart, brain and large blood vessels).

When thinking about the eye complications of diabetes, most people, including most health care professionals, think of *diabetic retinopathy*, the process through which the eye's light sensitive retina is damaged by chronic hyperglycemia. Indeed, diabetic retinopathy is arguably the most important example of diabetic eye disease, as it accounts for more than 22,000 cases of legal blindness each year in the United States, and more than 200,000 cases annually Worldwide. However, **diabetic retinopathy, which has several different forms and stages, is itself only one of several completely distinct types of diabetic eye disease.** Recognition and understanding of each of these particular types will help health care providers and patients alike to recognize specific eye and/or vision symptoms related to previously diagnosed diabetes and, perhaps, to suspect undetected cases of diabetes when a clinical diagnosis has yet to be made.

There are seven different **diabetic eye diseases:** diabetic cataract; glaucoma; diabetic keratopathy; diabetic optic neuropathy; diabetic cranial neuropathy; diabetic retinopathy; and retinal vascular occlusion. Each affects a different part of the eye, from the nerves that control eye movement to the nerve that connects the eye to the brain, from the front surface of the eye to its innermost internal layers. To better appreciate these various diseases, it will be helpful to conduct a "crash course" of sorts in ocular (eye) anatomy.

From there, we will explain the various kinds of diabetic eye disease, the treatments available for each and the things you can do to prevent or minimize vision loss from diabetes. Finally, we will consider the necessary elements of a thorough diabetic eye examination, including questions to ask your eye doctor and questions she should ask you, as well as some very important information about what to do if and when diabetic eye disease causes significant visual impairment.

Eyesight vs. Eye Health

It is extremely important that all diabetics understand a fundamental distinction between *good eyesight* and *good eye health*. The ability to see clearly (on an eye chart test or in the real world) is *not* equivalent to having healthy eyes. Many patients with serious eye disease have excellent eyesight, and the vast majority of patients who require eyeglasses or contact lenses to see clearly have healthy eyes. Just as for many patients with heart disease or cancer, patients with eye disease often have no symptoms at all until it is "too late." Regular, comprehensive eye examinations by an eye care professional (optometrist or opthalmologist) are the best way to ensure both good eyesight *and* good eye health.

Chapter Five:

Basics of Eye Anatomy

The eye is often compared to a camera, gathering light and forming images from the environment (the lens and shutter of the camera are analogous to the optical components of the eye —the cornea, iris and lens), developing those images onto an optical medium (the film inside a camera is analogous to the retina at the back of the eye), and producing a detailed pictorial/photographic representation of the environment (photographs are analogous to the electronic pictures that the brain receives from the retina). However, the eye is fantastically complex, much more so than any camera produced to date.

For example, there are two eyes, constantly in motion, which must be coordinated precisely to produce a three-dimensional, color image of the world. The eye is, of course, living tissue, which requires constant blood supply, nourishment and electrical input from the nervous system, processes which depend upon a myriad of biochemical substances and reactions, the complexity of which science is still attempting to fully understand. The eye must transform light energy into electrical energy and conduct that energy along the optic nerve to the brain where it is transformed again into an interpretable image of the world. The eye is also responsible for establishing and maintaining our circadian rhythm, our biological clock, which regulates much of our metabolism. Perhaps most remarkably, the eye does *all of these things all of the time.*

The **cornea** is the clear "window" at the front of the eye. It looks like the colored part of the eye but is actually transparent (the colored part is the iris, located *inside* the eye). The cornea has most (two-thirds) of the eye's focusing power, is composed of five distinct layers, has more nerve endings than *any* part of the body (just ask anybody who has been unfortunate enough to suffer a corneal abrasion), and has amazing regenerative powers provided its deeper layers remain intact. Inflammation or infection of the cornea is known as *keratitis*, while chronic disease of the cornea is called *keratopathy*.

Figure 5.1
External View - Ocular Anatomy

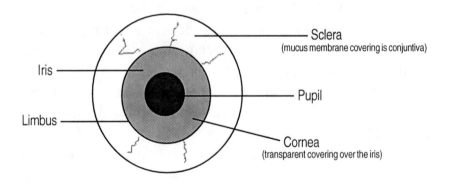

Iris
Limbus
Sclera
(mucus membrane covering is conjuntiva)
Pupil
Cornea
(transparent covering over the iris)

The **iris** is the colored (pigmented) part of the eye, and serves like the aperture stop on a camera, opening and closing to form a larger or smaller pupil to allow more or less light to enter the eye. The iris is contiguous with the major blood vessel layer of the eye, called the *uvea*, and also contains many nerves. Inflammation of the iris is known as *iritis* or *uveitis*.

The **sclera** is the white portion of the eye, and serves as a tough shell protecting the eye's internal parts. It is made of the same substances as the cornea, but lacks the latter's transparency. The sclera is covered by a clear mucous membrane called the *conjunctiva*; Inflammation or infection of the conjunctiva is called *conjunctivitis* (in laymen's terms, "pink eye").

The junction between the cornea and the sclera is called the **limbus**. Just below the limbus is a drainage canal (called the *trabeculum*) that drains internal fluid pressure (*aqueous humor*) out of the eye and back into the blood stream. Obstruction of this canal leads to a rise in internal eye pressure, a factor that can lead to glaucoma.

Figure 5.2
Cross-Section of Ocular Anatomy

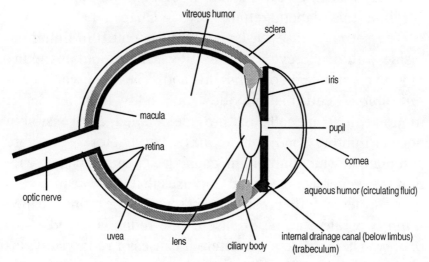

The **lens** of the eye is a transparent structure just behind the iris. It is about the size of an M&M candy piece, has one-third of the eye's focusing power, and serves to change focus from distance to near objects in persons under age 50. The lens is flexible (before age 50) and attached to a muscle (the ciliary muscle) that changes its shape and focusing power. Loss of lens transparency is known as *cataract.*

The **ciliary body** surrounds the lens, has muscles that alter the lens's shape and focusing power, and secretes filtered blood (called *aqueous humor*) into the eye that nourishes the cornea and lens (both of which are avascular — that is, contain no blood vessels to supply nourishment). Aqueous humor creates the eye's internal fluid pressure.

The **vitreous humor** is a transparent, gelatinous substance that fills the majority of the internal eye. It adheres to the retina and tends to liquefy over time, causing "floaters," specks or strands which many people notice in their vision, particularly when looking at a light colored background (e.g. a blue sky or a white wall.) Unfortunately, the vitreous humor provides a sort of lattice structure to which abnormal blood vessels may attach, as can happen in diabetic retinopathy (see "proliferative diabetic retinopathy" in Chapter 11).

The **retina** is a seven-layered transparent film lining the inside wall of the eye. It is highly vascular (contains many blood vessels), and contains rods and cones (known as *photoreceptors*), cells that provide vision in low light and detect motion (*rods*) and cells that provide detailed, color vision in normal lighting conditions (*cones*). The photoreceptors are stimulated by incoming light, causing a chemical chain-reaction that generates electrical impulses that are transmitted to the optic nerve. Inflammation or infection of the retina is called *retinitis*, while chronic disease of the retina is called *retinopathy*. There are several different causes of retinopathy, including high blood pressure, sickle cell anemia, arteriosclerosis (hardening of the arteries), lupus and other auto-immune diseases, certain medications/medical therapies (e.g. radiation treatment for cancer), and diabetes. The most posterior part of the retina, where incoming light is precisely focused to give good vision, is known as the *macula.*

The **uvea** is the blood vessel layer of the eye, sandwiched between the sclera and the retina. It is contiguous with the ciliary body and iris near the front of the internal eye, and serves to provide the outer layers of the retina with a blood supply and nourishment.

The **optic nerve** connects the eye to the brain, and is responsible for sending electrical impulses generated in the retina (by the rods and cones) to various parts of the brain for interpretation, and for receiving electrical impulses from the brain which control the eye's focusing muscles and pupil size. The optic nerve contains about one million individual nerve fibers, and has very limited ability to repair itself when damaged (like nerves throughout the body). Inflammation of the optic nerve is called *optic neuritis*, and chronic disease of the nerve is called *optic neuropathy*.

Movement of the eyeballs is controlled by six individual **muscles** attached to the sclera, each of which is controlled by a specific nerve (called *cranial nerves*) emanating from the base of the brain. Four of these muscles move the eyes horizontally (left or right), while another four move the eyes vertically (up or down). In addition, two of the six muscles rotate the eyes torsionally, that is, clockwise or counterclockwise. Disease affecting the nerves controlling these muscles is known as *cranial neuropathy*.

Key Points

1. **The eyes are connected to the rest of the body through the circulatory system & nervous system.**

2. **Any medical condition affecting these systems can affect the eyes.**

3. **Knowledge of eye anatomy allows better understanding of diabetic eye disease.**

Chapter Six:

Diabetic Cataract

Cataract is a clouding or opacification of the eye's internal lens, which is normally transparent. Lens opacities prevent light from focusing precisely on the retina. Common symptoms include loss of detail vision (like a smudge on the windshield of a car), reduced night vision, and increased sensitivity to glare. Some cataracts are very small and located at the periphery of the lens, away from the pupil, such that they have no impact upon a person's vision whatsoever. Other cataracts are quite large and/or located in direct line of the pupil (over what is called the *visual axis*), such that they dramatically reduce vision. The **features of a cataract that determine to what extent it will affect a person's vision** are, in decreasing order of importance: its precise *location* within the lens (opacities on the visual axis and those involving the posterior surface of the lens are the most bothersome); its *density* (dense cataracts allow less light to reach the retina and interfere with vision more); and its *size* (larger opacities interfere more than smaller opacities of equal density at any given location.)

World-wide, cataracts are a major cause of blindness. In the industrialized West, however, cataracts very rarely cause blindness, since they are nearly always surgically removable. Cataract surgery is typically a very quick (about 10-20 minute), painless, and quite safe procedure (the incidence of serious surgical complications is around 1%, an excellent percentage compared to many other kinds of surgery). **Cataracts occur as part of the normal aging process**, and by age 80, cataracts are virtually universal. **The mere presence of a cataract, though, does not in any way necessitate its removal**, as many cataracts have limited or no impact upon a given person's daily functioning, and they are typically *not* removed until they begin to interfere with a patient's *quality of life*.

Other than aging, cataracts are also caused by trauma to the eye (this often results in an instantaneous cataract, in contrast with the slow growing cataracts associated with "birthdays"), exposure to radiation (including ultraviolet rays from the Sun), certain medications including steroids (e.g. cortisone and prednisone), and certain metabolic/endocrine disorders like diabetes.

Diabetic cataracts are caused by hyperglycemia. Elevated blood glucose enters the eye via the aqueous humor (which is, essentially, ultra-filtered blood), and then enters the lens where it is converted into sorbitol, a form of modified glucose, which causes lens swelling and disorganizes lens proteins in such a way as to result in opacification (Figure 6.1). The lens consists of water, collagen fibers that are precisely arranged in a way that renders the entire lens *transparent*, and specific lens proteins that maintain this precise arrangement of collagen fibers. When sorbitol disrupts these lens proteins, thereby deranging (disorganizing) the lens fibers, diabetic cataract results. Blurry vision results almost immediately, but is often correctable with a change in eyeglass prescription. Eventually, enough transparency is lost such that changing glasses no longer helps.

Unlike virtually every other type of cataract, however, diabetic cataracts are **often reversible** if they are detected in time, and if blood glucose levels are normalized. Specialized cells within the lens are capable of pumping excess fluid out of the lens, reducing swelling and allowing lens fibers to regain their

Figure 6.1
Typical Progression of Diabetic Cataract

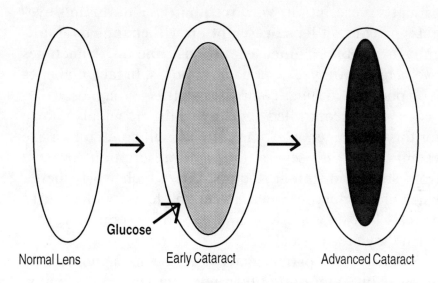

Normal Lens   Early Cataract   Advanced Cataract

Influx of glucose into the transparent lens causes fluid swelling and loss of transparency. Worsening causes permanent loss of transparency.

precise, optically transparent arrangement, provided the fibers have not been disrupted too severely or for too long a period of time. **Eye doctors are able to detect such cataracts at their earliest stages, before they cause permanent damage (opacity), and can counsel the patient and her diabetes doctor to reduce blood glucose levels as promptly as possible.** This is another important reason for all diabetics to have their eyes examined regularly.

Why Does My Eyeglass
Prescription Keep Changing?

One particularly fascinating and important aspect of the evolution of diabetic cataracts is the affect their development has on a diabetic's eyeglass prescription. Lens swelling (sometimes called *lenticular intumescence*) changes the optical power of the lens, which, in turn, changes the patient's prescription. **Very frequently, a diabetic's eyeglass or contact lens prescription will change dramatically as her blood glucose levels rise and fall**, sometimes over a matter of weeks, or days, or hours. In fact, diabetics with poor blood sugar control, as well as undiagnosed diabetics with uncontrolled hyperglycemia, are widely known for this phenomenon. Some patients will come for an eye examination with several different prescriptions in hand from several different doctors, one which works better when blood glucose levels are very high, one which works better when they are low, and one (or several more) for when they are "normal."

Some of these patients have never been diagnosed with diabetes but, more often than not, that is the explanation for their predicament. The prescription may become either stronger or weaker due to hyperglycemia (which direction it goes depends on what part of the lens swells with fluid). Patients who have never needed corrective lenses may find they rather suddenly need them, and patients who have always needed them may suddenly find they no longer do. **This can be very frustrating for both doctor and patient, but is always a sign of sub-optimal blood sugar control.** If the doctor looks closely, she can usually detect lens swelling and incipient cataract formation, or can refer the patient for blood tests to confirm a suspicion of diabetes when none has been previously detected. **Normalization of blood glucose at this point will stabilize the patient's prescription and stave off the formation of diabetic cataract.** This may take some time, but is always in the patient's best interest.

Surgical Treatment of Cataract

If diabetic cataract progresses to the point that irreversible opacity has occurred, then cataract surgery may be necessary to restore good vision. This is typically done with very small incisions and the use of sound waves to break up the cloudy lens, which is then removed and replaced with a clear lens implant (*intraocular lens*). At a later time, some patients may need a second procedure in which a laser is used to remove additional cloudy material that develops over the back surface of the implanted lens.

Cataract surgery has become the most frequently performed surgery in the US, and is also considered to be one of the safest. **The risk of complications from cataract surgery is higher for diabetics**, however. This includes possible infection (rare) and swelling of the retina causing reduced vision, called *cystoid macular edema* (common). Fortunately, there are treatments for each of these problems. Because proper healing after any type of surgery is aided by normal metabolism, including normal blood glucose levels, it is advisable that diabetics' blood sugars be normalized as much as possible prior to cataract surgery, as this reduces the risk of complications. Also, because cataract surgery can worsen any pre-existing retinopathy, **it is very important that retinopathy severe enough to require laser treatment is treated before cataract surgery, and that retinopathy not requiring laser treatment be monitored closely for progression following cataract surgery** (within 4-6 weeks after surgery).

<u>Key Points</u>

1. Cataract means loss of transparency of the eye's internal lens, causing blurred vision.

2. Cataracts are part of the normal aging process.

3. Hyperglycemia leads to premature cataracts by causing abnormal swelling of the lens.

4. Prior to cataract formation, diabetics' eyeglass prescriptions often fluctuate dramatically.

5. Diabetic cataracts are often reversible, if detected in time.

6. Cataract surgery safely and effectively 'cures' cataracts, but diabetics have a higher than average risk of post-surgical complications.

7. Good blood sugar control reduces the risk of both cataract and surgical complications.

Chapter Seven:

Glaucoma

Glaucoma is another kind of diabetic eye disease. Like cataracts, glaucoma occurs in many non-diabetics as well, but **diabetics are two to four times more likely to develop glaucoma than the general population.** Unlike cataracts, however, there is currently no cure for glaucoma, only treatment (in this way, glaucoma is very analogous to diabetes). Left untreated, glaucoma causes permanent vision loss and often results in blindness. The goal of treatment is to prevent or reduce vision loss as much as possible (just as with diabetes, the goal of treatment is to prevent or reduce complications). So what exactly is glaucoma?

Glaucoma is the term used to describe a *group* **of eye diseases that share the following characteristics**: *progressive, structural damage to the optic nerve, often but not always associated with an increase of internal eye pressure, resulting in a progressive and characteristic pattern of visual field (peripheral and then central vision) loss.*

As discussed previously, the optic nerve is responsible for sending electrical impulses from the retina to the brain. It consists of about one million individual nerve fibers that transmit visual information from distinct regions (*fields*) of the world that we see. Any damage to these nerve fibers results in fewer impulses and less visual information received. If enough fibers (between 30% and 50%) serving a particular field of vision are damaged, abnormal and permanent blind spots result (abnormal blind spot(s) are often referred to as *visual field defects* or *scotoma*, see Figure 7.1) Visual field defects are very subtle at first, and most people are quite unaware of them until severe vision loss has occurred. Glaucoma is the second leading cause of blindness in the US, with 1-2% of the population affected, and roughly 120,000 Americans are blind from the disease in 2002.

Figure 7.1
Normal and Abnormal Visual Field

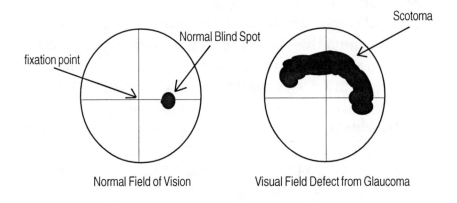

Normal Field of Vision   Visual Field Defect from Glaucoma

The most important test for uncovering glaucoma is examination of the optic nerve by use of one or several different lighted instruments that give the doctor a three-dimensional view of the shape and size of the nerve. This is best performed through an enlarged (dilated) pupil. The eye doctor evaluates the optic nerve for glaucomatous "cupping;" that is, structural deformation (physical damage) to the nerve (see figure 7.2).

The optic nerve typically looks like a bucket of vanilla ice cream viewed from above; *cupping* means the extent to which the "ice cream" (nerve) is "scooped out." In a normal eye, this cupping remains essentially the same throughout a person's life, whereas with glaucoma, the amount of cupping

Photograph 7.2
Optic Nerve "Cupping"

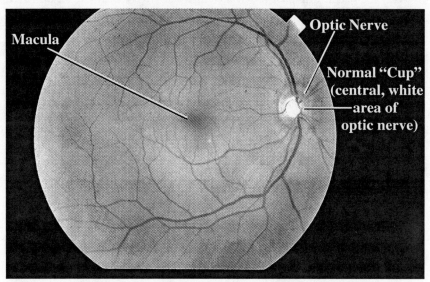

Normal optic nerve (right eye)

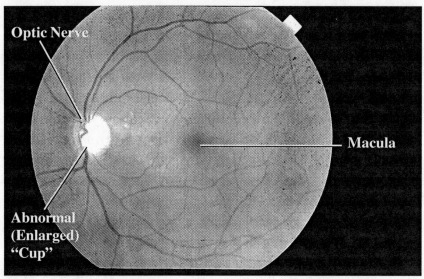

Glaucomatous optic nerve (left eye)

increases over time (usually one to several years — this is one good thing about glaucoma, it more often than not progresses slowly). At the earliest stages of glaucoma, it may take several years for damage to occur, and photographs coupled with computerized analysis of the optic nerves are often used to help the doctor assess any structural (cupping) change over time. If glaucomatous cupping is detected, a sophisticated test of peripheral vision, called a *visual field examination*, is done to demonstrate or rule out any visual field defects.

High Eye Pressure – Not the Whole Story

Internal eye pressure, called *intra-ocular pressure*, **is an important but often misunderstood element in the diagnosis of glaucoma.** Aqueous humor is continuously produced by the ciliary body, and must drain out of the internal eye to maintain a more or less constant level of internal eye pressure; the drainage canal (beneath the limbus) can become clogged or blocked for a variety of reasons, leading to a rise in intra-ocular pressure. Most cases of glaucoma are associated with (*not* necessarily *caused* by) elevated intra-ocular pressure, but some cases are not (between 5% and 20% of patients with definite glaucoma have eye pressures that fall within the "normal" range.) Furthermore, many people have intra-ocular pressure above the normal range (some well above normal) yet do not show any signs of optic nerve damage from glaucoma. **This is key; without optic nerve damage, there is no glaucoma.** In years past, high intra-ocular pressure was considered the necessary and sufficient cause of all glaucoma. We now know this is not true.

Some optic nerves are better able to tolerate elevated eye pressure than are others. For some optic nerves, even normal eye pressure is sufficient to cause damage. This variable tolerance of intra-ocular pressure is thought to be due to (1) genetic factors* and (2) the quality of circulation (blood flow) to the optic nerve, both of which vary from person to person. *This second factor may explain why diabetics are more susceptible to glaucoma,* as the micro- and macro-vascular effects of hyperglycemia, insulin resistance/ hyperinsulinemia and/or abnormal blood lipids impair the quality of circulation in many diabetics. Nonetheless, as a general rule, as the intra-ocular pressure rises, the *risk* of glaucoma (progressive optic nerve damage with visual field loss) rises as well.

A more rare form of glaucoma, called *neovascular glaucoma,* occurs when abnormal blood vessels block the internal drainage canal, and is much more common in diabetics. **Neovascular glaucoma in diabetics is usually found in conjunction with diabetic retinopathy**, is much more difficult to control, and requires laser treatment to the retina.

Aside from elevated intra-ocular pressure, the **risk factors for developing glaucoma** are: African-American ancestry (6-8 times the normal risk); family history of glaucoma, especially in siblings and parents (2-3 times the normal risk); age (most people with glaucoma are above 50); diabetes (2-4 times the normal risk); extreme nearsightedness (twice the normal risk); previous history of other eye disease, especially iritis or uveitis; sleep apnea (temporary stoppage of breathing while sleeping); previous history of migraine; unusually thin corneas.

Glaucoma is, then, a rather insidious disease with few or no symptoms until more than 1/2 of the optic nerve has been destroyed; **vision loss occurs gradually** in most cases. Glaucoma is best detected by a thorough eye examination which includes detailed three-dimensional examination of each eye's

---

A new genetic test for glaucoma, called "OcuGene," may signal which patients have a more aggressive form of the disease – one that worsens faster and is more resistant to standard medical therapy.

optic nerve, personal and family medical history to uncover any risk factors, examination of the eye's internal drainage canal, evaluation of each eye's visual field, photographic documentation of optic nerve structure*, and measurement of the intra-ocular pressure (a test called *tonometry*). Treatment is aimed at lowering intra-ocular pressure, as this has been shown to slow the progression of glaucoma even in cases where pressure was "normal" to begin with.

Treatment of Glaucoma

Current **treatments** to achieve this goal include medications, typically in the form of **eye drops**, which work by enhancing normal fluid (aqueous humor) drainage or by decreasing the amount of fluid produced by the ciliary body; **laser treatment** applied to the eye's internal drainage canal to enhance fluid drainage, or applied to the retina to treat neovascular glaucoma; **surgery** designed to allow internal fluid to drain to the external eye (sort of like poking a small hole in a water balloon.) Sometimes, a combination of these treatments is necessary, each of which has its pros and cons.

Most people diagnosed with glaucoma are treated initially with prescription eye drops, of which there are several different kinds. Of special interest to diabetics is the fact that one very effective type of eye drop medication, so-called **beta blockers, are known to mask the symptoms of *hypo*glycemia** in both Type 1 and Type 2 patients, and **tend to raise blood glucose levels** in Type 2 diabetics. Such *systemic side effects can be greatly reduced by merely closing the eyes for*

---

* New instrumentation uses an infrared laser to scan the optic nerve, creating a topographical map of its three-dimensional structure and surrounding optic nerve fibers, and allowing for detection (over time) of very subtle changes in optic nerve cupping due to glaucoma

three minutes following the instillation of beta blocker eye drops, as this helps prevent the medication from flowing into the tear drainage canal at the inner corner of the eyelid, and from there into the nose where it can be absorbed into the blood stream. Examples of beta-blocker eye drop medications include *Timoptic, Betoptic, Betagan, Cosopt, Ocupress* and *Optipranalol*. There are several other types of glaucoma drops that lower eye pressure without these potential effects. In addition, future treatment of glaucoma may include medications that improve blood flow to the optic nerve and/or fortify it against increased intra-ocular pressure.

Lowering Your Risk

Diabetics can reduce their risk of developing glaucoma by achieving and maintaining good blood sugar control, and by getting regular aerobic exercise in consultation with their diabetes doctors. In fact, several studies show that *aerobic exercise lowers intra-ocular pressure in addition to improving circulation,* both of which lessen the risk of glaucoma. The fact that aerobic exercise lowers blood sugar, burns fat, and improves cardiovascular health and overall well-being makes it an ideal preventative strategy for every person whose current health allows her to participate.

Beyond prevention, **diabetics can reduce their risk of losing vision to glaucoma by having their eyes examined regularly by a knowledgeable optometrist or ophthalmologist, and by getting and following through with treatment when indicated** (e.g. if eye drops for glaucoma are prescribed, take them as directed every day — just as with medical treatments for diabetes, medications don't work if they're not used consistently and correctly.)

Key Points

1. Glaucoma is a group of eye diseases that causes progressive damage to the optic nerve and a characteristic pattern of vision loss; it is the second leading cause of blindness in the U.S.

2. Diabetics are two to four times more likely to develop glaucoma than the general population, probably due to reduced eye circulation.

3. Internal eye pressure is one risk factor for glaucoma; other risk factors are black race, a family history of glaucoma, age, extreme nearsightedness, and diabetes.

4. Current treatment for glaucoma includes medications, laser treatment, and surgery.

5. If detected early and treated appropriately, the risk of blindness is greatly reduced.

Chapter Eight:

Diabetic Keratopathy

Diabetic keratopathy refers to the effects of diabetes on the cornea, the clear "windshield" at the front of the eye.** *Kerato-* comes from the Latin for "horn," as corneal tissue examined under the microscope reminded scientists of the microscopic appearance of horns from various non-human animals; -*Pathy* means illness or sickness (literally, "pathology"). Although not usually causing blindness, the corneal effects of diabetes can reduce vision and cause a great deal of patient discomfort and annoyance, and are often under-diagnosed in my experience.

The cornea is made up of five distinct layers. The outermost layer, the *epithelium* (rhymes with helium) contains many free nerve endings and adheres to the underlying tissue by specialized attachments (called *hemidesmisomes*). The innermost layer, the *endothelium* is responsible for pumping fluid (aqueous humor) out of the cornea as, like the lens, if the cornea swells significantly it loses its transparency. Chronic hyperglycemia affects both of these layers (figure 8.1).

Chronic hyperglycemia weakens the attachments between the epithelium and the underlying cornea, making diabetics more susceptible to (often very painful) corneal erosions, or loss of the surface layer of corneal cells. When this happens, nerve endings are exposed, and pain results. Most patients describe this as feeling like something is in the eye, with stinging and/or stabbing pain and extreme light sen-

Figure 8.1
Cross-Section of the Cornea

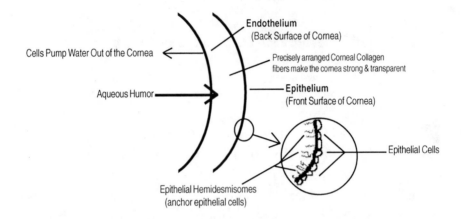

sitivity. Even simple blinking can cause such erosions to occur, and eye rubbing greatly increases the likelihood of such
an event. A similar phenomenon can occur in patients who
have experienced a traumatic corneal abrasion, especially from
fingernails and paper cuts, and in certain people with other
corneal diseases. Fortunately, the epithelium regenerates (re-
grows) very quickly, filling in any defects in a few hours or
days. Unfortunately, hyperglycemia delays the healing process, and newly grown cells may not attach any more firmly
than the original, poorly attached cells. This can lead to a
vicious cycle of erosions followed by healing followed by
more erosions (*recurrent corneal erosion syndrome*). Once
this cycle begins, acute episodes of high blood sugar can result in further erosions, even when overall blood sugar control is good.

Further complicating matters is the fact that **many diabetics have reduced corneal sensation**. This is essentially a form
of diabetic neuropathy affecting the corneal nerves (see "Diabetic Cranial Neuropathy" in Chapter 10). As a result, cor-

neal erosions may not be as painful as they would be for a non-diabetic individual, or they may not be felt at all. On the face, this may sound like a good thing — not having pain. However, pain is a good thing in that it tells us when something is wrong, so that we can discontinue whatever activity is causing the pain and/or seek medical advice (if you put your hand into a fire and it doesn't hurt, causing you to leave it in the fire longer, the well-being of your hand is in serious jeopardy!) Painless corneal erosions tend to worsen, and may progress to infection, corneal ulceration and permanent corneal scarring that affects vision. In the worst-case scenario, corneal scarring can cause blindness. Milder presentations are much more common, and *include symptoms* of scratchiness, grittiness, dryness and burning, if not outright pain. Chronic redness of the eyes is also common.

Treatments include the use of lubricating eye drops and ointments with varying degrees of viscosity, room humidifiers to increase moisture in the local environment, soft contact lenses which act like bandages over the damaged epithelium while still allowing vision, and topical antibiotics to treat or prevent infection. Sometimes, more aggressive laser or surgical treatments are used.

Chronic hyperglycemia also affects the ability of the endothelium to pump fluid out of the cornea. Aqueous humor circulating behind the cornea (see figures 5.2 and 8.1) naturally wants to seep into the cornea (in the lingo of fluid mechanics, the normally "dry" corneal tissue creates an *osmotic gradient*). The cells that comprise the endothelium act like miniature water pumps, preventing aqueous humor from seeping in beyond a minimal level. **If the cornea imbibes too much fluid, the precise arrangement of collagen fibers within the cornea is disrupted, causing a loss of transparency and a loss of clear vision** (similar to what happens with diabetic cataract formation). Excessive fluid build-up within the cornea can also result in very painful blister formation (called *bullae*) on the surface of the cornea. When the endothelial pump fails completely, the cornea loses all of its transparency and painful bullae are inevitable. Fortunately, this is not common.

There are several conditions which can cause the endothelial pump mechanism to fail: certain hereditary corneal diseases; trauma to the endothelium from intra-ocular surgery, including cataract surgery; inappropriate use of contact lenses, especially extended wear usage of lenses not designed for that purpose; certain metabolic diseases including *diabetes*. The pump works less effectively with age as well. *Total* failure of the endothelial pump is rare, and most cases involve relative failure and less than perfect pump function. **The most common finding in diabetic patients is a mild loss of corneal transparency that can affect one's** *contrast sensitivity*, the ability to discriminate subtler shades of gray from the background environment (as opposed to black on white — see figure 8.2). Diabetic retinopathy and cataract also can diminish contrast sensitivity. Various treatments include medications to dry out the cornea and, in severe cases, cornea transplant surgery.

Figure 8.2
Objects of Higher and Lower Contrast

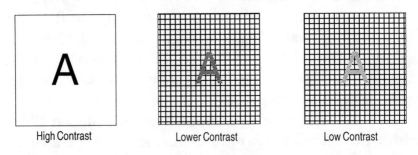

High Contrast   Lower Contrast   Low Contrast

A person with diabetic keratopathy affecting the endothelial "pump" might readily see the letter "A" in the first two boxes, but have difficulty seeing it in the third box

Reducing the Risk of Diabetic
Corneal Complications

The risk of diabetic keratopathy can be reduced by maintaining good blood glucose control, by wearing contact lenses conservatively (if at all) and with careful follow-up by an eye doctor on a regular basis, and by avoiding corneal trauma, including surgical trauma, unless necessary.

Diabetic patients frequently ask if they can safely wear contact lenses, and the correct answer is a qualified "maybe." Contact lenses pose a very low but serious risk to *all* patients, the risk of corneal infection with ulceration and permanent corneal scarring causing loss of vision (known as *ulcerative keratitis*). **Diabetics have a higher risk of ulcerative keratitis because of pre-existing keratopathy and reduced healing ability.** The decision to wear contact lenses needs to be made on an individual basis and in consultation with a knowledgeable eye doctor, but only in those who achieve and maintain good glycemic control, and only on a daily wear basis (i.e. no overnight wear of lenses).

What about refractive laser surgery? This miraculous technology has benefited many people who had been previously dependent on eyeglasses or contact lenses to see. Although this book is not intended as a treatise on the risks and benefits of procedures like LASIK (an acronym for "laser assisted intra-stromal keratomileusis") and PRK (another acronym for "photo-refractive keratectomy"), I will say that refractive laser surgery is absolutely terrific for some patients, and poses a very low but real risk of complications and/or undesirable side effects. **Some patients have a higher risk of problems**, however, including those with dry eyes, those with a previous history of corneal disease or autoimmune disease (e.g. ocular herpes, Sjogren's Syndrome, rheumatoid arthritis, and lupus), those with very large pupils or very thin corneas, and those with **diabetes**. This doesn't mean that diabetics cannot have this type of surgery, only that the *higher risk must be weighed against the benefits*. As with contact lens wear, only those with good blood sugar control and those without pre-existing keratopathy should consider this option.

Key Points

1. Diabetic keratopathy means chronic hyperglycemia has damaged the cornea.

2. Symptoms include a gritty sensation, pain, chronic redness, and loss of contrast.

3. Some diabetics have reduced corneal sensation, so discomfort may be minimal.

4. Diabetics must be cautious about using contact lenses and refractive laser surgery.

5. Good blood sugar control reduces the risk of diabetic keratopathy.

Chapter Nine:

Diabetic Ischemic Optic Neuropathy

O **ptic neuropathy refers to disease of the optic nerve**, and has a wide range of causes including infection, toxicity from prescription and non-prescription drugs (including consumed alcohol and tobacco), poor nutrition, inherited defects of nerve metabolism, glaucoma (see discussion above), multiple sclerosis, and poor circulation of the optic nerve. This last cause, lack of blood supply, is known as *ischemia* (see Chapter 3 for a general discussion of ischemia and the pathophysiology of diabetes.)

Ischemic optic neuropathy is an important cause of blindness and severe vision loss, particularly in people past 60 years of age. **The small blood vessels that deliver oxygen and nutrition to the optic nerve become blocked, resulting in a sudden, painless loss of vision in one eye**. This may be total or partial. In some cases, vision loss in the other eye may occur within hours or days,* in several months or years, or not at all. Ischemic optic neuropathy is really a stroke of the optic nerve. **Risk factors for this condition are the same as those for stroke: high blood pressure (hypertension), hardening of the arteries (arteriosclerosis), and *diabetes*. Persons with glaucoma also have a higher risk.**

---

* This happens with a particularly aggressive form caused by temporal arteritis, acute inflammation of the blood vessels in the patient's temples - immediate diagnosis and treatment with steroids can often prevent involvement of the second eye.

Diabetic ischemic optic neuropathy can occur in both younger and older patients, and in both Type 1 and Type 2 diabetics. **Because diabetes affects small blood vessels throughout the body, including those supplying the optic nerve, all diabetics are at risk, though the risk increases dramatically with age and the addition of other risk factors mentioned above.** When it occurs in younger, Type 1 patients, vision loss is usually less severe and often improves with time. In older patients, about 40% suffer severe loss of vision (20/200 or worse on the eye chart).

Unfortunately, there is no good medical or surgical treatment for this disease once the initial event and damage have occurred. Protecting the involved eye from future attacks and the uninvolved eye from *any* attacks by reducing risk factors is the best recourse. If both eyes (or the better seeing eye) are affected, consultation with a low vision specialist will help maximize any remaining vision potential (see Chapter 15 for a discussion of "Low Vision.") **The risk of diabetic ischemic optic neuropathy can be reduced by controlling hypertension, improving one's blood lipid profile through diet, exercise and medication, not smoking, taking aspirin (in consultation with your physician) and maintaining optimal blood sugar control.** Like stroke, this is one condition where prevention is the best medicine.

Key Points

1. This condition is essentially a stroke of the optic nerve.

2. Vision loss is sudden (unlike most types of glaucoma) and painless (like most types of glaucoma).

3. Good blood pressure, blood lipid, and blood sugar control lower the risk of this condition.

Chapter Ten:

Diabetic Cranial Neuropathy

This is yet another variation on diabetic neuropathy. The nerves affected in this condition are those that control the muscles both inside and outside the eye, as well as sensation (pain) from the cornea. **These nerves originate at the base of the brain, and are called "cranial nerves."** There are actually twelve distinct pairs of cranial nerves (each member of the pair connects to one side of the body or the other), five of which serve the eyes; the other seven serve the ears, nose, throat, tongue and face. Each pair of cranial nerves is designated by a Roman numeral, I through XII. **Lack of adequate blood supply (ischemia) to any one or combination of these nerves results in loss of function, either movement or sensation** (when *movement* is lost, the condition is sometimes referred to as "nerve palsy"). **Because diabetes and hyperglycemia affect the small blood vessels providing oxygen and nutrition to each of these nerves, diabetics have a much higher risk of experiencing cranial neuropathy than the general population.**

Cranial Nerve II is the *optic nerve*, the nerve responsible for sending visual information to the brain, neuropathy of which is discussed in some detail in the previous sections on glaucoma and diabetic ischemic optic neuropathy. Here, we will consider other cranial neuropathies affecting the eyes.

Cranial Nerve III controls the *internal* ocular muscles responsible for regulating *pupil size* and *focusing* from far to near, *four of the six extra-ocular muscles* which allow us to move the eyes, in unison, inward, upward, downward, and extorsionally (that is, rotating them clockwise or counterclockwise outward, away from the nose), and *the muscle which keeps our eyelids open*. Cranial Nerve III has a lot of jobs, and neuropathy involving it has a profound impact on vision: **the eyelid becomes droopy or closed** (a condition called *ptosis*); **the pupil is often (but not always) fixed and dilated** (enlarged and unresponsive to light); **the focusing (ciliary) muscle is often (but not always) paralyzed; the eye is unable to turn either upward, downward, or inward.** The affected eye turns/wanders down and out, away from the nose.

When the eyelid is open (or manually *held* open), **double vision results** (both vertical and horizontal). This is because single vision, using the two eyes together (what is commonly called *binocular vision*) requires both eyes to be *precisely coordinated* and pointing at the same object at the same time. Any condition disrupting this precise coordination causes more or less severe double vision (called *diplopia*). **Diabetes is a leading cause of "Third Nerve Palsy."**

Cranial Nerve IV controls the single extra-ocular muscle responsible for turning the eyeball downward when the eye is simultaneously turned inward, and for turning the eyeball intorsionally (that is, rotating it clockwise or counterclockwise inward toward the nose.) This nerve is quite thin and fragile, and is prone to damage from even minimal head trauma or shaking, as well as the microvascular effects of chronic hyperglycemia. Palsy of this nerve causes **vertical double vision that** can sometimes be eliminated by tipping the head to the shoulder opposite the damaged nerve. The affected eye turns/wanders up and rotates out.

Cranial Nerve V is the trigeminal nerve, responsible for movement of the jaw, and sensation from the face, nose and eye. This large nerve has three divisions (branches); **the "ophthalmic division" regulates sensation and pain from the**

cornea. **Neuropathy affecting this division results in a loss of corneal sensation, and greatly increases the chance of diabetic keratopathy** (see Chapter 8). This same division is linked to Cranial Nerve VII (called the *facial nerve*, neuropathy of which is called *Bell's Palsy*), one of the functions of which is to produce moisture from the tear gland, a reason why many patients with trigeminal neuropathy, including diabetics, also suffer dry eye.

Cranial Nerve VI controls only one eye muscle, the one that allows the eyeball to turn outward, away from the nose. Palsy of this nerve results in **horizontal double vision**, which can sometimes be reduced or eliminated by turning the head to the side of the damaged nerve. The affected eye turns/wanders inward (toward the nose).

Each of these cranial neuropathies can be caused by a variety of underlying conditions, including neurological diseases (e.g. multiple sclerosis), brain tumors and aneurysms, stroke, head trauma, heavy metal poisoning, and diabetes. **Cranial neuropathies, especially those causing double vision, are not an infrequent initial symptom of previously undiagnosed diabetes.** The mere presence of one (or more) of these neuropathies in a diabetic patient, however, does not exclude other causes. Only thorough evaluation by a trained health care provider can establish a definitive cause, which, in some cases, cannot be determined with absolute certainty. **Diabetic patients, in particular, can reduce their chance of cranial neuropathy by optimally controlling blood sugar, high blood pressure, and abnormal blood lipids.**

Fortunately, neuropathy of Cranial Nerves III, IV and VI, the ones controlling eye muscle movement and causing double vision, usually resolves on its own without treatment. This typically takes between 1 and 3 months but can take up to 6 months. As double vision is often extremely disconcerting and disabling, many of these patients prefer to patch one eye, which immediately resolves the problem.

If bothersome double vision persists beyond six months, a *prism* prescription can be included in the glasses prescription to eliminate or reduce that double vision (prism moves the world as seen by one or both eyes to a different position — in effect, if one eye is unable to move in a certain direction because of a weakened or paralyzed nerve and muscle, prism moves the world to where that eye *can* move.) Prism can be used sooner, but will often have to be changed or removed from the prescription as the affected cranial nerve recovers. Surgical correction of affected muscles is also an option in some cases, after a minimum of six months recovery.

Key Points

1. **Diabetic cranial neuropathy is nerve damage affecting sensation from the cornea and/or the control of eye muscles.**

2. **Loss of eye muscle control typically causes double vision.**

3. **Double vision usually resolves over several months.**

4. **Good blood pressure, blood lipid, and blood sugar control reduce the risk of this condition.**

Chapter Eleven:

Diabetic Retinopathy

Diabetic retinopathy is perhaps the single most important cause of adult blindness in the Western World, and **almost 15% of all blindness in the United States is caused by diabetic retinopathy**. This statistic takes on added economic significance when we consider the fact that many of these cases occur in younger adults who are often in the prime of their income earning years.

Diabetic retinopathy, unfortunately, is a very insidious disease. It usually causes no symptoms in its earliest, most treatable stages, and by the time symptoms are noticed, many patients have experienced irreparable damage and/or loss of vision, and the overall prognosis is poorer. **This is why dilated eye examinations by an experienced and knowledgeable eye doctor are so vital. The earlier retinopathy is detected, the more can be done to prevent, or at least delay, significant loss of vision**.

The retina lines the inside surface of the eye, like wallpaper covering a wall. It has seven distinct layers, each with unique characteristics and functions, which are readily observable under a microscope. In the clinical setting (i.e. the eye doctor's office), the individual layers are not all directly observable, but a variety of examination tools and techniques, combined with intimate knowledge of retinal anatomy, allows the eye doctor to examine the layers damaged by diabetes, to make a diagnosis and evaluate the type and severity of diabetic retinopathy, and to make treatment recommendations. Such recommendations may include observation over time, improved blood sugar control, laser treatment of the retina, use of prescription medications, surgical treatment of the retina, or a combination of these.

The Normal Retina

The normal retina contains many blood vessels. Large arteries coming from the neck (the carotid arteries) branch off into smaller arteries serving the eye (the ophthalmic and ciliary arteries) which branch off into smaller arterioles coursing through and beneath the retina (retinal and uveal arteries, respectively) which branch off into thousands of microscopic capillaries designed to deliver blood to each bit of retinal tissue (see photograph 11.1). Veins return blood to the heart.

Diabetic retinopathy alters this normal anatomy and its function in several distinct steps or stages, each of which has

Photograph 11.1
Normal Retina and Optic Nerve

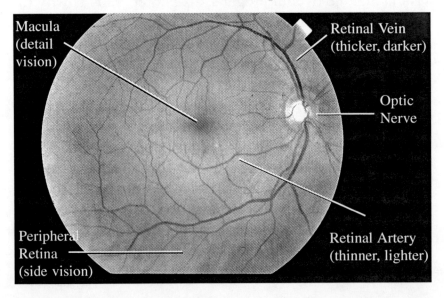

Macula (detail vision)

Retinal Vein (thicker, darker)

Optic Nerve

Peripheral Retina (side vision)

Retinal Artery (thinner, lighter)

its own characteristics. The earlier stages are less worrisome, but may progress to the vision-threatening, advanced stages unless something intervenes (whether that something is better blood sugar control, blood pressure control, laser treatment, luck, or some other factors that have yet to be fully understood.) Here, we will consider the stages of retinopathy.

Background Retinopathy

In a pattern that we are familiar with now, **hyperglycemia damages these smallest, most fragile blood vessels, the capillaries, by disrupting their internal lining and allowing blood, serum and other blood components to leak** out (sort of like poking pin holes in a running garden hose from the inside out.) When examining the retina, a doctor can see small amounts of blood (called *dot and blot hemorrhages*), abnormal out-pouchings of the capillaries (called *micro-aneurysms*), and chalky, whitish deposits from leaking lipid (blood fats) and protein (these deposits are called *hard exudates* — they are similar to water deposits left on a bath tub). The severity of this condition ranges from mild (e.g. a few micro-aneurysms or dot hemorrhages) to severe (e.g. numerous micro-aneurysms and hemorrhages throughout the retina combined with many hard exudates.) As long as most of these changes occur outside of the macula, the central part of the retina responsible for good, detail vision, patients usually will have no symptoms at this stage of retinopathy, often called "Non-proliferative Diabetic Retinopathy" (see photograph 11.2)

Photograph 11.2
Background/Non-proliferative
Diabetic Retinopathy

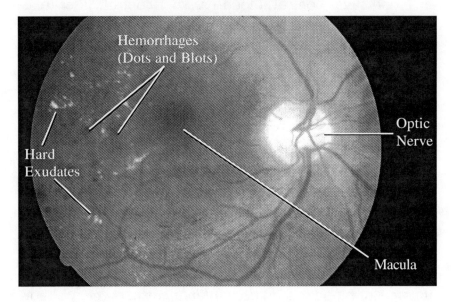

<u>Pre-Proliferative Retinopathy</u>

At this stage of diabetic retinopathy, capillaries have become damaged to the point that they close off (*capillary non-perfusion*), such that **retinal tissue is receiving inadequate blood supply to meet its needs** (*ischemia*). The retinal veins, which take blood out of the eye, develop irregularly shaped segments (called *venous beading*), some capillaries develop tiny, abnormal fronds which are thought to be precursors to new blood vessel growth (these are called IRMA — an acronym for "intra-retinal microvascular abnormalities"), and patches of retinal tissue begin to die, causing the formation of wispy white areas on the retinal surface (called *cotton wool spots* due to their appearance). Retinal hemorrhages and hard exudates may or may not be severe at this stage.

As with "Background Diabetic Retinopathy," patients typically will not have any symptoms as long as the macula remains relatively uninvolved (see photograph 11.3).

Photograph 11.3
Pre-Proliferative Diabetic Retinopathy

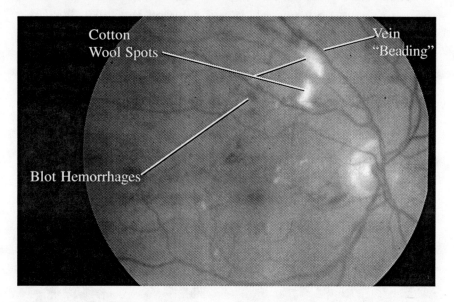

Proliferative Diabetic Retinopathy

This is the most serious stage of retinopathy, as it often leads to blindness if undetected and/or untreated. Dying retinal tissue releases chemical messengers that stimulate the cells to **grow (proliferate) new blood vessels on the surface of the optic nerve and retina**. At first blush, this sounds like a "good" thing — the body trying to grow a new system of blood vessels to replace the old, damaged system. Unfortunately, these new blood vessels, called *neovascularization* (neo- meaning "new" and -vascularization meaning "blood vessel growth"), are quite *abnormal*.

First, they grow on the surface of the retina, not in the deeper layers where the normal blood vessels are found, and where the retinal tissue is most in need of more blood supply. Second, **these new blood vessels are very fragile**, much more so than normal retinal blood vessels, and have a tendency to break and **bleed profusely**. Unlike the original, damaged retinal capillaries which leak only small amounts of blood *within* the retina, the new vessels bleed a lot on the *surface* of the retina and *into* the clear gelatin which fills the inside of the eye, the vitreous. **This vitreous hemorrhage very often (but not always) will interfere with a person's vision**, appearing as a veil, a cloud, or streaks of red material (photograph 11.4).

Photograph 11.4
Proliferative Retinopathy
with Vitreous Hemorrhage

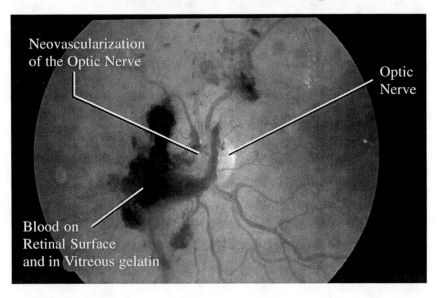

If severe enough, vitreous hemorrhage will result in almost total loss of vision. Fortunately, the blood will often clear, over a period of weeks or months, and vision may return.

However, the abnormal, new vessels may (and usually do) continue to grow and bleed. This pattern of new blood vessel growth and bleeding leads to **the development of fibrous scar tissue attached to the new vessels, the retina and the vitreous**. Bleeding causes the gelatinous vitreous to contract, pulling on the abnormal vessels (causing more bleeding) and the retina, literally tearing the retina off the back wall of the eye (very much like wall paper coming off, or detaching, from a wall.)

This process is known as **"traction retinal detachment"** (because the complex of scar tissue and blood vessels has resulted in traction, tugging on the retina, causing it to detach — see photograph 11.5). When the retina detaches from the blood vessels beneath it (the blood vessels of the uvea), it begins to die quickly, resulting in total blindness. A detached retina may be surgically reattached, but the adherence of fi-

Photograph 11.5
Proliferative Retinopathy
with Traction Retinal Detachment

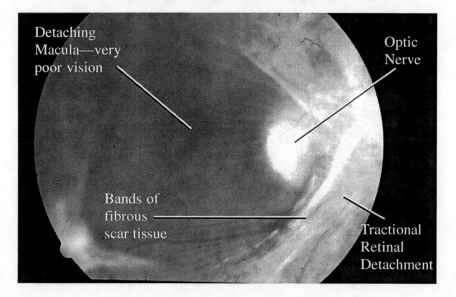

Detaching Macula—very poor vision

Optic Nerve

Bands of fibrous scar tissue

Tractional Retinal Detachment

brous scar tissue and poor health of the retina make this quite challenging, and visual results are often not good.

Diabetic Macular Edema

There is yet another type of diabetic retinopathy, distinct from the stages detailed above, "Diabetic Macular Edema." This can occur either alone, or in conjunction with the other types of retinopathy, and is **the major cause of vision loss in diabetics, with more than 100,000 new cases per year.** Serum leakage from blood vessels surrounding the macula causes the macula to swell with fluid (edema), and may result in the formation of "hard exudates" (see photograph 11.6). Either one of these processes interferes with the sharpness of incoming light, which the cornea and lens are designed to focus precisely on the macula, and damages the retinal photo-

Photograph 11.6
Diabetic Macular Edema

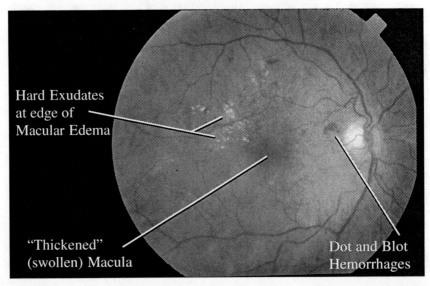

Hard Exudates at edge of Macular Edema

"Thickened" (swollen) Macula

Dot and Blot Hemorrhages

receptors (primarily "cones"), resulting in loss of clear vision and reduced ability to see colors. If the photoreceptors become too damaged, irreparable loss of vision to the point of legal blindness (but not complete blindness) results. High blood pressure is known to accelerate diabetic macular edema, as do elevated blood lipids and cigarette smoking.

Treatment of Diabetic Retinopathy

It is important to know that the **treatment of diabetic retinopathy is based upon a great deal of clinical research involving many thousands of patients and using various treatment strategies**. The "Diabetic Retinopathy Study" (DRS), the "Early Treatment of Diabetic Retinopathy Study" (ETDRS) and the "Diabetic Retinopathy Vitrectomy Study" (DRVS) are three of the most important studies used to guide the recommendations made to individual patients.

For **background retinopathy,** patients typically are advised, in consultation with their regular diabetes physician, to achieve better blood glucose control, especially as shown by their glycosylated hemoglobin (HbA1c) test results, to control any high blood pressure and improve blood lipid profiles (through diet modification, exercise and medication), and to quit smoking. Depending upon the severity of the retinopathy, patients will be seen by the eye doctor every 4 to 12 months.

Patients with **pre-proliferative retinopathy** will also be asked to improve glycemic control, blood pressure and lipids, and cease smoking. Occasionally, laser treatment of the retina may be recommended to prevent imminent new blood vessel growth (neovascularization). These diabetics need to be followed very closely for the development of vision-threatening proliferative retinopathy, every 2 to 6 months.

For **proliferative retinopathy,** the current gold standard of treatment is "pan-retinal photocoagulation" (often called

PRP), **laser treatment** applied to much of the retina, not just the areas of new vessel growth ("pan-retinal" meaning "across the entire retina," "photo-" meaning "using light energy," as in laser, and "coagulation" referring to forming blood clots within retinal tissue.) This amounts to a series of laser burns, created outside of the macula, which have the effect of halting the proliferation of new, abnormal blood vessels, as well as causing the regression of existing neovascularization.

With PRP, abnormal blood vessels themselves are *not* specifically targeted but, rather, retinal tissue itself. Why does this work? Although several explanations have been offered, most experts believe that laser burns destroy (kill) enough tissue to *decrease the retina's overall demand for adequate blood supply,* thereby turning off the release of chemical messengers that cause neovascularization in the first place. **With less retinal tissue to need oxygen and nutrients provided by the blood stream, there is less need for new blood vessels to meet that need.** The "Diabetic Retinopathy Study" showed that PRP reduces the risk of (permanent) serious vision loss (20/800 or worse on the eye chart, with glasses) by 50-75%.

Because proliferative retinopathy is highly correlated with diabetic kidney disease, these patients must have their kidney function monitored closely, and be treated accordingly (of course, this should be happening independently of eye examinations anyway.) **As improved blood glucose and high blood pressure control lower the risk of worsening retinopathy (and kidney disease) over time, all reasonable steps should be taken to optimize these factors as well.**

Pan-retinal laser treatment does have some side effects. Because laser is applied to the peripheral parts of the retina, **peripheral (side) vision is often reduced.** Moreover, because the peripheral retina contains mostly rods, the retinal cells responsible for giving us vision in low light conditions (e.g. at night or in a darkened room), **most patients report a definite decrease in night vision abilities** after PRP. Laser treatment **may also increase vitreous hemorrhage, which**, as discussed above, can greatly reduce vision but often clears on its own within 6 months (if it doesn't, the blood can be surgically removed by vitrectomy). Even with these negative effects, though, PRP is still the mainstay of treatment for proliferative retinopathy, as it cuts the risk of severe vision loss by more than half.

In addition, new techniques are on the horizon for treating proliferative retinopathy, including drugs that block the chemical pathways causing growth of new blood vessels. For example, a substance called "vascular endothelial growth factor" (VEGF for short) is produced by the body and is required for the development of retinal neovascularization. Drugs capable of inhibiting VEGF (aptly named *VEGF inhibitors*) may someday make PRP obsolete, provided they are shown to be safe and effective.

Patients unfortunate enough to have developed a **traction retinal detachment** as a result of proliferative retinopathy will almost always require a **vitrectomy** surgery, where the gelatinous vitreous gelatin filling the majority of the eye is removed, along with as much of the fibrous scar tissue that caused the retinal detachment as possible. The retina may then be reattached using a variety of techniques including additional laser treatment, freezing of torn retinal edges, placement of a scleral buckle (a band placed around the sclera which "squeezes" the detached retina up against the underlying tissue), and infusion of air bubbles or silicone oil to hold the retina in place. The risk of re-detachment is often high in these cases, and multiple surgeries are sometimes required.

Patients with **diabetic macular edema** (DME) are divided into two categories: those with and those without *"clinically significant* macular edema." The characteristics of "clinically significant" macular edema have been well defined by the *Early Treatment of Diabetic Retinopathy* study (ETDRS), and are memorized by every eye doctor in training. These characteristics have to do with the exact size and location of macular swelling. "Clinically significant diabetic macular edema" is much more likely to cause severe loss of vision than is macular edema that is not "clinically significant." **The ETDRS showed that focal laser treatment, laser burns applied directly to areas of the macula where leaky blood vessels are causing swelling, reduces the risk of severe vision loss by about 50% in diabetics with clinically significant macular edema.**

Patients who do not have "clinically significant" swelling did not benefit sufficiently from laser therapy in the study, but these patients need to be watched carefully for worsening edema that requires future laser treatment. As with PRP treatment for proliferative retinopathy, focal laser treatment for macular edema has some side effects, most notably the creation of central blind spots that may or may not affect a given person's visual functioning (for example, these new blind spots can cause patients to lose their place more often while reading text.)

New drug and surgical therapies for DME currently are being tested, including implantation of time-release steroid medications within the vitreous, and use of so-called *PKC inhibitors*, chemicals designed to "waterproof" leaky blood vessels that serve the macula.* **All patients with diabetic macular edema are advised to improve blood sugar and**

---

*Just prior to publication of this book, a study by a multinational team of researchers has found that a lipid soluble form of Vitamin B1 (thiamine) prevented the development of diabetic retinopathy in rats over a 36-week period. The synthetic thiamine derivative, called _benfotiamine_, has been used safely for more than a decade in Europe, where it is prescribed to treat painful neuropathies. Benfotiamine boosts levels of a cellular enzyme called *transketolase* by 300-400%, a factor that prevents hyperglycemia from forming chemical compounds known to damage the cells lining the inner walls of blood vessels, including both AGEs (see p. 129) and PKC. Naturally occurring Vitamin B1 (thiamine) is water soluble, and boosts transketolase levels by a mere 20%. Because benfotiamine is lipid (fat) soluble, a fact that undoubtedly increases its retention within the body and its effectiveness, its potential toxicity also is increased (just as Vitamin A, a lipid soluble substance, is healthful in moderation but harmful in excess). Clinical trials to determine safety and efficacy in humans are expected to begin within the next year.

blood pressure control, improve blood lipid levels (lower total cholesterol, triglycerides and bad LDL cholesterol, and elevate good HDL cholesterol), and cease smoking.

Does Snoring Worsen Retinopathy?

New research suggests that obstructive *sleep apnea* is a significant risk factor for the development and worsening of all forms of diabetic retinopathy. People suffering from this condition cease breathing for short periods of time while sleeping due to physical obstruction of the upper airway; loss of normal muscle tone around the pharynx (wind pipe) allows the pharynx to collapse when inhaling air, a problem often but not exclusively caused by obesity. Typical symptoms include snoring, restless sleep and excessive daytime sleepiness. It is thought that decreased levels of oxygen in the blood stream of patients suffering from this condition leads to retinal hypoxia (oxygen starvation) and retinal edema (swelling), both of which are aggravating factors for diabetic retinopathy.

The Benefits of Good Diabetes Control for All Types of Diabetic Retinopathy

Research has clearly shown that intensive diabetes management, including lowering blood glucose and blood pressure levels, greatly reduces the risk of getting diabetic retinopathy, and slows down its progression (worsening) in patients who do have it. **In fact, the DCCT showed that a 10% reduction in HbA1c reduces the risk of retinopathy progression by 43%, while the UKPDS showed that better control of blood pressure reduced the risk of worsening retinopathy by up to 34%.**

Many experts believe that retinal capillaries are damaged when blood glucose levels approach 180 mg/dl on a consistent basis (this is equivalent to a HbA1c of 8.0%.) This is why most guidelines recommend that patients strive to keep their average blood glucose at or under 150 mg/dl (equivalent to an HbA1c of 7.0% or less.) To achieve these targets, **patients should perform regular home blood glucose tests and adjust their diet, exercise and medications accordingly. They should also work closely with their doctor to find the right medications and dosages, perform quarterly glycosylated hemoglobin tests, and monitor their blood pressure and blood lipids.**

After having diabetes for 10 years, 60% of patients will have at least the beginning stages of retinopathy; after 20 years, that number jumps to more than 90%. This underscores the general rule that the longer a person has diabetes, the greater is the chance of having complications. **The best way to detect diabetic retinopathy is through regular, dilated retinal exams, the importance of which cannot be over-emphasized in early treatment and prevention of vision loss.**

Why is dilation so important? Because it allows the eye doctor to see **more of the retina, more easily, and in 3-D** (a fact that is especially critical in detecting diabetic macular edema and retinal detachments, as well as optic nerve changes due to glaucoma.) Once diabetic retinopathy is detected, patients then can receive the optimal treatment based upon the findings of the DCCT, the UKPDS, the DRS, the ETDRS, and the DRVS.

The Limits of Clinical Research: Populations versus Individuals

It is important for all patients to realize, however, that **no treatment strategy is perfect in all cases,** and that even treatments that have been scientifically proven to significantly reduce the risk of vision loss may not prevent vision loss in *particular* cases. This is because **risk reduction statistics**

apply to entire populations, not to specific individuals. So, for example, if a particular laser treatment has been proven to reduce the risk of serious vision loss by 50%, this number applies to the large group of people studied — the risk of serious vision loss for the entire group, considered as a single unit, was reduced by 50%, but *individual* risk was not necessarily reduced by this amount. In fact, to continue with this example, some of the diabetics studied may have had an 80% reduction in risk, while some may have had only a 20% reduction. Unfortunately, some diabetics lose their vision even after receiving the absolute best treatment, or doing everything the doctor has recommended.

Individual risk reduction cannot be assessed with statistical or scientific certainty because particular individuals are unique; even for medical studies of identical twins there are only 2 subjects, a completely inadequate number for scientifically/statistically assessing the benefit of a specific medical treatment. Researchers are often fond of saying their results can be "generalized to entire populations," but this does not mean they can be generalized to *any given individual*. **We may say that research results apply to unique individuals, *all things being equal*, but, as it turns out, all things are never equal.** Variations in environment and genetics always make a difference from one person to the next. Well done clinical research definitely applies to "all of us," but not necessarily to "each of us."

Are, then, the results of scientific research beneficial to unique individuals? (beneficial to *each* of us, in addition to being beneficial to *all* of us?) The answer is yes. To the extent that human beings share a common biology, a common genetic make-up, and a common environment (and this is, beyond all doubt, *a large extent*), each of us will have a high probability of a favorable response to a medical treatment that has been proven effective for a large population of us. The results of clinical research are vi-

tally important, and following recommendations generated by such research is *smart*, because we are stacking the odds in our favor. It doesn't guarantee each of us success, but it does *maximize our chances*.

Many patients with diabetes do, unfortunately, suffer vision loss. Sometimes that vision loss is mild; sometimes it is severe. Medical, surgical and laser treatments do not always improve vision; very often, they only stabilize it, and sometimes they provide no demonstrable benefit. In such situations, patients should be referred to, or seek out on their own, **Low Vision services which will help them to maximize whatever remaining vision potential they have. There is always something that can be done to help visually impaired patients**, whether they have modest vision loss or are totally blind. Getting help is a matter of knowing where to look for it — knowledge is power (see Chapter 15 for a discussion of "Low Vision.")

Key Points

1. Retinopathy is *the* leading cause of vision loss in diabetics, and a leading cause of blindness.

2. Diabetic retinopathy occurs in several different forms or stages.

3. Chronic hyperglycemia damages the blood vessels of the retina, leading to serum leakage, deposits of lipid and protein, and hemorrhaging; eventually, lack of adequate blood supply may cause growth of new, abnormal blood vessels, which break easily and bleed profusely. Fibrous scar tissue develops and, ultimately, detaches the retina.

4. Retinopathy may cause *no* symptoms unless the macula is affected or vitreous bleeding occurs.

5. Treatment of retinopathy includes improved blood sugar, blood pressure, and blood lipid control; retinal laser treatment is used when retinopathy threatens vision, and reduces the risk of severe vision loss by 50-75%.

6. The risk of retinopathy increases over time; research shows that tight blood sugar and blood pressure control each significantly reduce the risk.

7. Sleep apnea may worsen retinopathy; diabetics who snore or who are obese should be evaluated for the possibility of this condition.

8. Annual dilated eye examinations are the best way to detect retinopathy at its earliest, most treatable stages.

9. Following recommendations based upon research stacks the odds in your favor.

Chapter Twelve:

Other Retinal Diseases Associated with Diabetes

Aside from diabetic retinopathy, there are several other distinct retinal diseases that are more often associated with diabetes, though they certainly can occur in non-diabetics as well.

Hypertensive retinopathy, damage to the retina from chronic and/or acutely elevated blood pressure, leads to abnormal narrowing and **stiffening of the retinal arterioles, serum, lipid and protein leakage in addition to bleeding from retinal capillaries, and even swelling of the optic nerve**. Vision is not usually affected unless the macula becomes involved or optic nerve swelling impairs the transmission of electrical signals to the brain. Because diabetics have a greater than average tendency for high blood pressure (twice the normal risk), their risk for hypertensive retinopathy is also greater.

Like arteries and veins throughout the body, retinal arteries carry blood *from* the heart and lungs *to* the retina, while retinal veins carry blood *away* from the retina *back* to the heart and lungs. Retinal blood vessels, arteries and veins, travel together throughout the retina and *cross over* one another as they deliver and remove blood. Because high blood pressure causes stiffening of the retinal arteries (just as a flimsy garden hose becomes stiffer, or more rigid, when the water pressure is increased), **these arteries have a tendency to crimp (push on, deform) the less rigid veins where the two cross**

over one another. This can cause a dramatic, localized narrowing of the vein that impairs (decreases) blood flow (Figure 12.1).

Figure 12.1
The Mechanics of Hypertensive
Retinopathy and Vein Occlusion

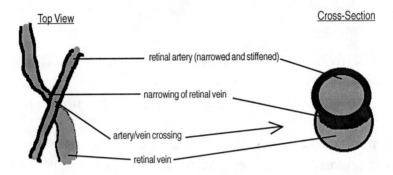

Top View   Cross-Section

retinal artery (narrowed and stiffened)

narrowing of retinal vein

artery/vein crossing

retinal vein

~ The increased rigidity of the artery compresses ("crimps") the less rigid vein. This causes reduced blood flow and allows platelets to form a clot, which can block (occlude) the vein

In addition, if platelets in the blood stream (cells responsible for normal clotting) clump together within this narrowed area of a retinal vein, a tendency which is increased by both slower blood flow and any increase in the adherence (stickiness) of platelets, a "thrombus" (blood clot) forms which may completely block (occlude) the vein. **Occlusion of a retinal vein** results in substantial bleeding, swelling (retinal edema) and tissue damage; if a vein supplying the macula is affected, or if vitreous bleeding or edema affect the macula, at least some vision is lost. As with diabetic retinopathy, ischemia (lack of blood supply) to surrounding retinal tissue may occur, which can lead to profound vision loss, as well as the formation of **new, abnormal blood vessels** (*neovascularization*) **and neovascular glaucoma**, both of which can cause blindness.

Because many diabetics tend to have stickier platelets, and because of a greater likelihood of high blood pressure, diabetics have a much higher than average risk of retinal vein occlusion (about 60% of patients who suffer retinal vein occlusion have diabetes, high blood pressure, or both.) However, the culprit in this form of diabetic eye disease is not hyperglycemia per se (as with all the other eye diseases discussed in this section), but hypertension, possibly coupled with an abnormal clotting tendency. **Visual impairment from retinal vein occlusion ranges from none to severe**, depending upon which vein is blocked (the central vein supplying the entire retina versus one of the smaller branch veins supplying only a portion of the retina), to what extent the macula is involved, and the development of complications like retinal neovascularization and neovascular glaucoma (these often take several months to develop).

Vision loss due to macular edema, or neovascularization, both can be helped or stabilized with laser treatment (just as with diabetic retinopathy). **Diabetics' risk of retinal vein occlusion can be decreased by keeping blood pressure and blood glucose levels normal, by not smoking, and by taking a daily baby aspirin** (in consultation with a physician). Detection of symptom-free retinal vein occlusion, and any hypertensive retinopathy that often precedes it, depends upon getting **regular dilated eye examinations.**

Finally, diabetics also have a higher risk of **retinal artery occlusion**, due to their higher chance of abnormal blood lipid profile and arteriosclerosis (hardening of the arteries). Cholesterol plaques may break off the inside wall of the carotid artery in the neck, travel to the ophthalmic artery or smaller arteries within the retina and become lodged there. Partial blockage may cause symptoms of foggy vision or temporary loss of vision (lasting a few seconds to a minute) in one eye, due to reduced blood supply and oxygen starvation. Total blockage results in death of retinal tissue and **sudden, pain-**

less loss of vision, which may be partial or total. This disease is essentially a stroke of the retina. Immediate medical treatment helps some patients, but is often unsuccessful. **Diabetics can reduce their risk of retinal artery occlusion by knowing and improving their blood lipid profile, by controlling blood pressure and blood sugar, and by not smoking.**

Key Points

1. **Diabetic retinopathy is not the only serious retinal disease for which diabetics are at risk.**

2. **Hypertensive retinopathy, retinal vein occlusion, and retinal artery occlusion also put diabetic patients at risk for severe vision loss.**

3. **Good blood pressure, blood sugar, and blood lipid control reduce the risk of these diseases.**

Chapter Thirteen:

My Recommendations for Preventing and Minimizing Diabetic Eye Disease

The common themes throughout this entire section on the prevention and treatment of Diabetic Eye Disease have been:

•**Keep blood sugar levels as close to normal as possible through proper diet, exercise, and medication, in consultation with a physician knowledgeable about diabetes care**

Chronic hyperglycemia plays a direct role in the development of six of the seven types of diabetic eye disease, from cataract to glaucoma to keratopathy to ischemic optic neuropathy to cranial neuropathy to retinopathy. Because hyperglycemia negatively affects blood lipids, including the increased adhesiveness of platelets, it also plays an indirect role in retinal vein and artery occlusion. I have never had a diabetic patient with a consistent HbA1c of less than 7.0% suffer severe vision loss from diabetic retinopathy. Conversely, I have seen many patients lose their vision when HbA1c values are consistently above 9.0%. **A diet low in simple carbohydrates (refined sugar, white bread and rice, and almost all packaged snack foods) and high in complex carbohydrates (whole grains, fruits and vegetables) helps prevent large swings in blood sugar levels**, as these complex carbohydrates are converted into glucose more slowly, giving the body more time to "catch up." Such foods are said to have a **low** *glycemic index*.

Exercise works beautifully to lower blood sugar independently of insulin levels, makes insulin work more effectively, lowers internal eye pressure, and improves circulation to all parts of the body, including the eyes. Exercise and proper nutrition together can help obese and overweight diabetics lose excess weight, and even modest weight reduction can greatly improve glycemic control. Perhaps most importantly, **regular aerobic exercise lowers the risk of cardiovascular disease better than virtually every other preventative measure.** Simply walking briskly, 20 minutes a day, five times a week, would be of tremendous benefit to most diabetics. However, **your diabetes doctor should always be consulted before starting any exercise regimen** (see *Side Bar* on *Exercise and Diabetic Retinopathy*).

Many different medications are now available to lower blood sugar, and many more are being developed. Keeping in regular contact with your physician will help you enjoy the benefits of the "latest and greatest" in medical treatment and control your blood sugar optimally. Ideally, diabetics would control hyperglycemia without medications. For some patients though, it is not possible (including virtually all Type 1 patients and most Type 2 patients.) **Good blood sugar control is far more important in the long run than the hassles of finding and taking the right diabetes medications.**

•Check your blood sugar levels at home on a regular basis, and know your HbA1c values

Speaking of good blood sugar control, **how do you know if you have good control?** Unfortunately, a good number of patients do not. Regular glycohemoglobin testing reveals the average blood sugar over an 8-12 week period, but says noth-

A Word About Exercise and Diabetic Retinopathy

Some health care professionals and diabetes educators caution patients with diabetic retinopathy to refrain from exercise that might aggravate retinal bleeding. For example, it is sometimes stated that patients with retinopathy should avoid jarring exercise that requires rapid head movement (for instance, basketball or kick boxing), or exercise requiring muscular strain that might elevate blood pressure (for instance, weight lifting), as these activities are said to increase the likelihood of retinal bleeding.

Although there is merit in being cautious, it is important for patients to understand that such restrictions concerning exercise and retinopathy apply to neither the majority of diabetics, nor even to the majority of patients with diabetic retinopathy. In fact, **the only group of patients at risk for retinal bleeding associated with exercise are those with untreated, recently treated or actively bleeding proliferative diabetic retinopathy, as these patients have abnormal blood vessels that *can* be broken quite easily.** There is absolutely no reason that people with non-proliferative retinopathy (background or pre-proliferative) or those with successfully treated proliferative retinopathy cannot participate in vigorous physical activity, including moderate resistance (weight) training, as fragile new blood vessels (neovascularization) either do not exist or have regressed following laser therapy.

Certain forms of physical activity may aggravate cardiovascular disease or diabetic neuropathy, so patients should always check with their regular diabetes doctors about their favorite forms of exercise, especially before beginning any *new* exercise program. As for retinopathy, the key point is to know what stage of retinopathy you have, and to ask your eye doctor specifically about the risks, if any, of your exercise regimen.

ing about day-to-day fluctuations, the measurement of which allows patients to adjust their diet, exercise and medications to normalize their *daily* blood glucose levels. Regular home blood glucose testing is very important for precisely this reason and, in my view, should be performed each and every day. **In combination with HbA1c measurements, daily (sometimes multiple) home blood sugar testing gives the best overall picture of, and plan for, how well you are controlling your diabetes.**

Interestingly, some studies have shown that increased frequency of home blood glucose testing does not necessarily result in better HbA1c values. Some people believe this shows that home testing is not that important. To the contrary, **I believe this proves that patients are either not using or are not being given the necessary information and tools by their health care providers to adjust their treatment regimen according to their home blood sugar readings.**

If a home reading is high, patients must be instructed by their doctors (and their assistants) *exactly* how to respond. For those on insulin therapy, a sliding scale is convenient (i.e. if a home blood glucose reading is above a certain level, the patient is instructed to take a certain number of *extra* units of insulin.) For those not using insulin, a temporary modification of oral medication dosage and/or dietary intake (for example, counting and adjusting carbohydrate intake) and/or activity level (more or less exercise) allows patients to react immediately to high (or low) blood sugar readings, and *will* result in better HbA1c values!

Patients of mine often tell me that they "know" what their blood sugar levels are without testing them, that they can "feel" whether or not they are "low or high." Research has shown that long-term diabetics *lose* their ability to sense *hypo*glycemia, and small studies have suggested that patients are not all that good at predicting their own blood sugars, but **I was curious to determine just how accurate patients' own predictions are on a**

large scale, so I conducted a study of 148 consecutive diabetics seen for eye examinations in my own office. Patients were asked to make their best prediction about their current blood sugar levels, and were then tested by means of a blood glucose meter. The results: 81% of diabetics were off by more than 50mg/dl; 44% were off by more than 75 mg/dl; 28% were off by more than 150 mg/dl; Patients were twice as likely to estimate too low as too high; Type 1 diabetics (18 of the 148 patients), on average, were only slightly worse "guesstimators" than Type 2 diabetics. **The bottom line — patients are very poor at predicting their blood glucose levels.** As the DCCT and UKPDS showed that even modest (10-20% reductions) in HbA1c values dramatically reduced the likelihood of diabetes complications, the value of measuring home blood glucose levels and acting on them to reduce HbA1c levels becomes even more clear.

•Check and control even mild high blood pressure through proper diet, exercise and medication, in consultation with your diabetes doctor

The UKPDS clearly showed that, for Type 2 diabetics at least, controlling hypertension lowers the risk of retinopathy and retinopathy progression even more than does tight blood glucose control; in addition, it significantly reduces the risk of macro-vascular disease (heart disease, stroke and peripheral vascular disease.) It is thought that **elevated blood pressure makes the smallest blood vessels leak more blood and serum** by causing damage additional to that caused by chronic hyperglycemia, and **reduces circulation to the retina and cranial nerves, including the optic nerve**.

Restricting excessive sodium intake (by limiting high salt foods like canned soups and meats, cheese, and many snack foods) helps the kidneys to maintain a normal blood pressure. Losing excess weight also reduces blood pressure. Regular, aerobic exercise lowers blood pressure by releasing chemicals that dilate (enlarge) peripheral blood vessels (thereby reducing resistance to blood flow and, hence, blood pressure.) Many types of blood pressure medicines are available. One type, **the so-called "ACE-inhibitors," reduces blood pressure in the kidneys and has been proven to prevent and even reverse early diabetic kidney disease**.

•Check and improve your blood lipid profile with the same

Abnormal blood lipids (high cholesterol, triglycerides and LDL, and low HDL) increase the risk of blood vessel occlusion (blockage), thereby increasing the risk of glaucoma, ischemic optic neuropathy and other cranial neuropathies, retinal artery occlusion, and diabetic retinopathy. **In particular, diabetic macular edema is often much worse in patients with lipid problems**.

Reducing dietary consumption of fats, especially saturated fats (any type of fat that is solid at room temperature - butter, margarine, animal fat, shortening - and any packaged foods containing partially hydrogenated fats) will help combat hardening of the arteries (*arteriosclerosis*) and atheroma formation (*atherosclerosis*). Consumption of foods containing omega-3 fatty acids, a type of fat that thins the blood and is associated with a lowered risk of cardiovascular disease, may also be beneficial (salmon, sardines, flax seed), as is dietary fiber. For an excellent discussion of fats and dietary/lifestyle changes that lower the risk of vascular disease, I highly recommend a book by Andrew Weil, M.D. entitled *Natural Health, Natural Medicine,* as well as the groundbreaking book by Dean Ornish, M.D.

entitled *Dr. Dean Ornish's Program for Reversing Heart Disease*.

Both weight loss and aerobic exercise combat atherosclerosis and arteriosclerosis by lowering triglycerides and LDL while raising HDL. Exercise and weight reduction also improve blood glucose control, a factor which itself improves blood lipid abnormalities. Finally, a host of medications are available to improve blood lipids if dietary and lifestyle changes prove inadequate.

Of particular interest to diabetics is a recently published study conducted by the *National Academy of Sciences* comparing the effects of food ***preparation*** on the likelihood of arteriosclerosis and cardiovascular disease. It was conclusively shown that foods prepared my *baking, roasting or broiling* (high temperature preparation without the use of water) are significantly more prone to produce certain chemicals thought to damage blood vessels than are identical foods prepared by *boiling or steaming* (slower rise in temperature with the use of water).

This phenomenon is due to toxic, inflammatory substances, called *AGEs* (an acronym for "advanced glycation end products") that result from the combination of sugars and proteins in prepared foods, and are formed at a much higher rate when foods are cooked at high temperatures without water. AGEs stay in the body a long time, and were already believed to play a role in the development of diabetes complications (from eye disease to kidney disease to heart disease) as a result of chronic hyperglycemia, which encourages their formation in body tissues *independently* of food preparation methods.

Although this recent study does not prove that people who eat baked, broiled, roasted and/or micro waved foods suffer long-term vascular (or any other) complications, it does show that chemicals associated with vascular disease are present at much higher levels in both the foods and bodies of persons who eat foods prepared this way. The strong implication for diabetics, of course, is that we should reduce the formation of AGEs both by maintaining tight blood glucose control *and* by cooking foods more slowly with water (boiling or steaming) as much as possible.

•If you smoke, quit

Smoking constricts blood vessels throughout the body, especially the smallest blood vessels, including those that serve the retina and optic nerve. This **reduces the amount of blood flow and raises blood pressure, both of which greatly increase the risk of diabetic eye disease**. Nicotine also reduces the ability of red blood cells to carry oxygen, thereby promoting hypoxia (oxygen starvation), which further increases the risk of eye disease. Smoking promotes the production of "free radicals," chemical compounds that damage cells; this is thought to be one of the reasons smokers develop cataracts at a younger age than non-smokers, and that *smokers are 2-3 times more likely to develop macular degeneration, the leading cause of legal blindness in the Western World.*

•See an optometrist or ophthalmologist for a dilated eye examination each year (see Chapter 14 for a description of what a thorough diabetic eye exam should include), and more often if your eye doctor recommends it

Most cases of serious vision loss from diabetes are preventable with early diagnosis and timely treatment. Dilated eye examinations greatly increase the chances of early diagnosis. The three most common causes of significant vision loss in diabetics are: cataract, retinopathy, and glaucoma.

Each of these is treatable, and the first of these is essentially curable (with surgery). **Good vision on an eye chart does *not* mean there is no diabetic eye disease, as many patients with severe retinopathy and glaucoma have 20/20 vision at the time of diagnosis.**

Diabetic keratopathy does not typically cause severe vision loss, is treatable, and somewhat reversible (with improved blood sugar control.) Diabetic ischemic optic neuropathy is not treatable and only sometimes reversible; fortunately, it is less common than other types of diabetic eye disease. Cranial neuropathy causing double vision does not cause permanent vision loss, and usually improves on its own; however, it is a sign of poor circulation and poor blood sugar control, both of which increase the risk of retinopathy, retinal vein occlusion, glaucoma, optic neuropathy, keratopathy and cataract.

Here are a few more pearls of wisdom that will help you prevent or minimize the effects of diabetes on the eyes:

•Take a daily multivitamin and an additional 800 IU of Vitamin E, and ask your doctor about the risks and benefits of taking a coated baby aspirin daily

Hyperglycemia and large swings in blood sugar are thought to generate free radical chemical compounds that damage ocular tissue (in fact, free radicals are thought to play a role in many diseases throughout the body.) Vitamins and other compounds in the foods we eat act as free radical "scavengers;" that is, they chemically neutralize the damaging effects (called *oxidation*) of free radicals (for this reason, they are called *anti-oxidants*). Because many of us fail to eat the right balance of foods to protect us from free radicals, and because many diabetics have reduced ability to absorb micro-nutrients (including anti-oxidants) from the foods they eat, **taking a daily multivitamin is a reasonable strategy and poses minimal risk**. I recommend additional Vitamin E because it appears to promote blood flow in addition to its anti-oxidant properties, and several studies have suggested that it reduces the risk of heart disease.

The benefits of aspirin therapy have to do with the fact that diabetics have stickier platelets (the part of blood that allows us to form blood clots.) Because of this, diabetics have a higher risk of forming atheromas, the blood vessel plaques found in atherosclerosis. Aspirin makes the platelets less sticky, and research shows it lowers the risk of heart attack and stroke in diabetics with pre-existing atherosclerosis.

The ETDRS proved that aspirin therapy does not cause diabetic retinopathy to worsen, and some people believe it improves circulation to the eye and lowers the risk of retinal vein and artery occlusion, glaucoma and ischemic optic neuropathy (although in patients with active vitreous hemorrhage, from proliferative diabetic retinopathy or retinal vein occlusion, avoiding aspirin until most of the blood has cleared may still be prudent if the bleeding is interfering with vision.) Some individuals, of course, cannot take aspirin due to allergy, ulcer or other condition causing internal bleeding, or poorly controlled high blood pressure.

A number of additional supplements and botanical medicines are thought to help stabilize or normalize blood glucose levels, including *inositol, quercitin, chromium, alpha lipoic acid, Gymnema sylvestre* (a native Indian plant long used as a treatment for diabetes in that country), *bitter melon* juice, *fenugreek, bilberry* (European blueberry) and *salt bush*. Some multivitamin supplements specifically formulated for diabetics contain at least some of these ingredients. You might wish to try experimenting with the use of these naturally occurring substances in consultation with a naturopathic physician experienced with diabetes; for an excellent discussion, including results of clinical research and recommended dosages, see the *Encyclopedia of Natural Medicine* by Michael Murray, N.D. and Joseph Pizzorno, N.D.

•If you have poor blood sugar control, and try to improve it with a sudden increase in aerobic exercise, see the eye doctor 3 months after the start of your new regimen

I make this recommendation from both personal and clinical experience. When glycemic control is poor and suddenly improves, oftentimes retinopathy appears, or worsens in patients with pre-existing retinopathy (for example, non-proliferative retinopathy abruptly becomes proliferative retinopathy.) This is referred to as **the re-entry phenomenon** ("re-entry" because blood sugar levels re-enter a more normal range after being abnormal.) Aerobic exercise exacerbates this phenomenon, perhaps because retinal tissue that is receiving barely enough blood supply to function has added stress placed upon it by exercise, or because the additional blood supply that exercise promotes encourages the retina to deliver that supply by growing new (unfortunately abnormal) blood vessels.

•Reduce stress as much as possible

Stress causes widespread changes throughout the body. **It causes the release of epinephrine (adrenalin) that constricts blood vessels and raises blood pressure. Stress triggers the release of glycogen by the liver, which, in turn releases glucose and raises blood sugar.** Both of these processes affect diabetes control and the likelihood of diabetes complications, including eye complications. Of course, it's easy to tell someone to reduce her stress levels, and more difficult to actually do it. I'll be the first to admit that this is one aspect of good diabetes management that I often fail at miserably. The reason I fail, I believe, is because I fail to practice stress reduction strategies *consistently*.

What are some stress reduction strategies? A partial list might include: regular aerobic exercise, meditation, avoidance of caffeine and other stimulants, yoga, biofeedback techniques, massage therapy, playing relaxing music, and various breathing techniques. The list could go on and, I'm sure, would include unique and effective strategies for unique individuals. **The point is to be aware of the importance of stress reduction, to avoid the trivial triggers of stress, and to find some activities that foster relaxation and engage in them on a regular basis**.

> **•Seek out health care professionals who are knowledgeable, communicate effectively and serve as your advocates**

This is perhaps one of my fuzzier (more esoteric, less easily definable) recommendations, but one of the most important. **Knowledge is power, and you want a health care team with plenty of both.** You, the patient, also must strive to be knowledgeable, because it will empower you to make educated health care decisions, to be your own advocate, and to find top-notch health care professionals. A book by Irl Hirsch, M.D., entitled *12 Things You Must Know About Diabetes Care Right Now!*, provides an excellent framework for asking your doctors the right questions, and for knowing what answers you should expect.

Effective communication means that members of your health care team should explain your diagnosis, available treatments and prognosis in a way that you can understand, and that you feel free and are encouraged to ask questions and actively participate in the management of your diabetes. Of course, the more educated you are about diabetes, its treatments and its complications, the more sophisticated will be your questions and your doctors' answers to those questions.

Effective communication also means that members of your health care team communicate with each other. This is very important, because diagnoses and treatments made by one doctor may very well affect recommendations made and treatments offered by other doctors. Your eye doctor, for example, should send timely reports to each of your other doctors and health advisors, whether they be a general practitioner, an internist, an endocrinologist, a nephrologist, a cardiologist, a neurologist, a podiatrist, a diabetes educator, a dietician, a pharmacist, or all of these. It is also important that your eye doctor receive reports from your other doctors and advisors, or at least a summary of their findings and recommendations compiled by your primary care physician. If your doctors don't specifically say they will send their findings to your other doctors, **ask them to do so**.

Because diabetes is a chronic medical condition, and good care requires frequent visits to members of your health care team, **it is important that all members truly serve as your advocates**, that they encourage you, that they praise your successes and sympathize with and constructively address your failures, **that they work with you and each other in your best interest, and that you always feel they are "on your side."** This is what good health care professionals do, and if one of yours does not, find another. There are too many excellent doctors and health advisors to settle for less.

Key Points

1. Keep blood sugar levels as close to normal as possible through proper diet, exercise and medication, in consultation with a physician knowledgeable about diabetes care.

2. Check your blood sugar levels at home on a regular basis, and know your HbA1c values.

3. Check and control even mild high blood pressure through proper diet, exercise and medication, in consultation with your diabetes doctor.

4. Check and improve your blood lipid profile with the same.

5. If you smoke, quit.

6. Have a dilated eye examination each year, more often if specifically recommended.

7. Take a daily multivitamin and an additional 800 IU of Vitamin E, and ask your doctor about the risks and benefits of taking a coated baby aspirin daily.

8. If you have poor blood sugar control and try to improve it with a sudden increase in aerobic exercise, see the eye doctor 3 months after the start of your new regimen.

9. Reduce stress as much as possible.

10. Seek out health care professionals who are knowledgeable, communicate effectively and serve as your advocates.

Chapter Fourteen:

What To Expect From an Eye Examination

Now that we have considered the various kinds of diabetic eye disease, the treatments available for each, the results of clinical research, and some recommendations for avoiding or minimizing eye complications, let's discuss **the elements of a thorough diabetic eye examination**. It is unlikely that any two eye doctors (or any kind of doctors) will conduct an examination in exactly the same way; procedures, techniques and explanations that work well for one health care provider may not work for another, and vice versa. Here, it is simply my aim to describe and explain the fundamentals of an eye exam that will allow you to ask the right questions and assess the thoroughness of your examination experience.

All eye examinations should start with a detailed **case history.** The doctor will ask about any particular eye or vision problems that you are experiencing, your general and ocular health, any medications that you are taking, any drug allergies, whether or not you smoke, and the medical history of your blood relatives. **Patients often ask why so much general health information is required for an eye examination, and the answer is really quite simple: because the eyes are connected (via the blood stream and nervous system) to every part of the body, and because the eyes and vision are affected by many general health conditions, medications, and genetic influences that are shared by or inherited from your family members.**

Diabetics, in particular, should be asked about how long they have had diabetes (date of diagnosis), the specific medications they are using for diabetes treatment, the previous diagnosis of any diabetes complications (eye, kidney, nerve or vascular), the frequency and range of home blood glucose readings, the most recent home reading, and the results of their last glycosylated hemoglobin test. As we have seen in previous chapters, the answers to these questions will give the eye doctor a good sense of overall diabetes control and the likelihood of finding eye complications. **The patient's responsibility is to know the answers to these very important questions**.

After conducting a case history, the patient is typically asked to **read the eye chart** wearing any corrective lenses previously prescribed. This is not a test, nor anything to be embarrassed about if the letters are unclear. Guessing is absolutely allowed, as the true definition of "visual acuity" is the smallest letters that can, *just barely*, be identified correctly. The results allow the doctor to gauge just how far off the prescription might be, or the effects of any eye diseases (cataracts, diabetic retinopathy, keratopathy, to name just 3 of many possibilities) that will be uncovered in subsequent parts of the eye exam.

A test of stereopsis (stereo vision, or the ability to see three-dimensionally) may be given, which precisely measures depth perception and helps evaluate how well the two eyes work together. **Color vision testing** also may be performed. In my experience, this is an important test, as academic research (including a study in which I participated while in optometry school) shows that diabetic retinopathy can cause a specific kind of color vision defect (in lay terms, "color blindness"). In fact, some researchers believe that subtle, acquired color vision deficiencies may precede the earliest stages of diabetic retinopathy by months to years.

The patient's **pupil reactions** should be evaluated by shining a bright light into each eye. This checks the neurological integrity of the connections between the optic nerve and the brain, and many optic nerve diseases (including advanced glaucoma and ischemic optic neuropathy) may be first detected this way. Many diabetics are found to have sluggish pupil responses, and this suggests some degree of (so-called "autonomic") neuropathy affecting part of Cranial Nerve III (see Chapter 10 on "Diabetic Cranial Neuropathy.") The patient also is asked to **follow a moving target** with her eyes only, which allows the doctor to evaluate the function of the six extra-ocular muscles and assess any possible double vision from nerve palsy.

A test of peripheral (side) vision may be given, which may be as simple as detecting the number of fingers the examiner is holding up, or as sophisticated as a computerized visual field test which more precisely determines how good the patient's peripheral vision is in relationship to thousands of other patients. All patients, diabetics included, should have their peripheral vision checked by professional examination regularly, as **visual field loss can be very subtle until severe damage has occurred** (as in glaucoma).

At some point, the patient will be **"refracted,"** the process through which a new eyeglass prescription is determined ('tell me which lens choice is better, choice #1 or choice #2'). No part of an eye examination is probably more frustrating to patients than this test; oftentimes, neither of the two choices is clear, or both choices look identical. Take heart — this is entirely normal; the test *intentionally* forces the patient to pick between crummy choices or choices that look virtually the same. Also, no one answer counts very much at all. The examiner is looking for *consistency* and will show you the same choices repeatedly (even though you may not be aware of it!) When the test is completed, the prescription almost always is correct, and vision will be as clear as the patient is capable of seeing. If the doctor is a sub-specialist, such as a retina or glaucoma sub-specialist to whom your regular eye doctor has referred you, refraction may or may not be done (see the following section on *Types of Eye Doctors*).

Several points about refraction should be of particular interest to diabetic patients. As discussed in Chapter 6, changes in blood sugar can have a dramatic impact upon your prescription, so it is important that you and the doctor know if your overall blood sugar control is good (as reflected by recent HbA1c testing), and if your blood sugar level the day of the eye exam is high, low or relatively normal (as reflected by home blood glucose testing that day). **Dramatic prescription changes may be the result of poor glycemic control, which should be corrected before getting a new eyeglass or contact lens prescription.**

Diabetics sometimes have more difficulty than usual discriminating between the various choices presented during refraction. This may be due to loss of contrast sensitivity from keratopathy, cataract, or retinopathy (I personally prefer to perform a specialized test of contrast sensitivity on all diabetics.) Large decreases in nearsightedness, or large increases in farsightedness, especially in one eye more than the other, are often signs that the patient has diabetic macular edema and should alert the patient and doctor to this possibility.

All patients should have their eyes examined by a **slit lamp,** a specialized microscope that gives the examiner a highly magnified view of the eyes. The patient places her chin on a chinrest, and a bright (slit of) light is shined on various parts of the eye, including the cornea and conjunctiva, the iris, the lens, the anterior (most forward part) of the vitreous, the tear ducts and the eyelids. This allows the doctor to detect any sign of diabetic **cataract** (see Chapter 6), **keratopathy**, abnormal blood vessel growth on the iris (the cause of **neovascular glaucoma** — see Chapter 7) or blood cells that might signal **vitreous hemorrhage** (see Chapter 11). A fluorescent dye may be dabbed into the eyes, which is especially useful for detecting keratopathy of the corneal epithelium (see Chapter 8). Measurement of internal eye pressure (**tonometry**) also may be performed with this instrument, a similar hand held device, or a machine that blows a puff of air at the cornea. Examination of the eye's internal drainage canal, with a specialized, mirrored contact lens, also is performed at the slit lamp microscope.

Eye drops should be placed into the eye, which **dilate the pupils.** Drops typically take 15 to 30 minutes to work, cause blurred vision and make patients more sensitive to light. Once the pupils are dilated, the internal eye is examined once again with the slit lamp microscope, very powerful hand held lenses or other instruments which allow the doctor to **visualize the posterior vitreous, optic nerve and retina in considerable detail.** A combination of techniques and instruments is often used to ensure completeness. Use of the slit lamp microscope to view the retina and optic nerve is very important, because the doctor is able to use both of her eyes to **examine the patient in stereo (3-D), a feature which is critical for assessing diabetic macular edema, as well as optic nerve cupping from glaucoma.**

The eye doctor may recommend other tests depending upon the patient's particular diagnosis, including retinal or optic nerve photographs to document baseline findings and subsequent changes, more sophisticated visual field testing, or a retinal dye test called "fluorescein angiography" (a fluorescent dye is injected into the vein of a patient's arm, and travels to the blood vessels of the retina which are photographed, allowing the doctor to evaluate retinal circulation.) After all tests have been completed, the eye doctor should explain her findings and treatment recommendations to the patient in understandable detail, and ensure the patient's questions are answered. Sometimes, the patient may be referred to an ophthalmic sub-specialist for further evaluation (see *Types of Eye Doctors* on next page).

At the conclusion of the eye exam, every patient should know her diagnosis, be informed of various available treatment options as well as the doctor's recommended treatment plan, the prognosis for her condition, and exactly when she should have an eye examination again. This may sound confusing, but may be as simple as telling the patient, for example, that she is nearsighted (*myopic*), that possible treatments include eyeglasses, contact lenses, or refractive surgery, that the doctor recommends eyeglasses for this patient's particular case, that the nearsightedness will most likely increase over time, and that her eyes should be re-examined in two years.

For the diabetic patient, the same basic format should be followed, with special emphasis on those findings pertaining to diabetic eye disease. The doctor should discuss the need for prescription lenses, including any changes in prescription, particularly as those changes relate to diabetic cataract or retinopathy. The patient should be advised as to the presence or absence of any eye muscle abnormalities due to diabetic cranial neuropathy, as well as the presence or absence of diabetic keratopathy, cataract, glaucoma or other optic neuropathy, and retinopathy or other retinal abnormality.

If diabetic eye disease (or any eye disease) is detected, the doctor's recommendations and treatment plan should be explained in detail (written instructions are ideal, though not always possible), **the next appointment date should be established** (always one year or less) and **a letter describing the patient's eye exam findings should be sent promptly to each of her doctors. All of the patient's questions should be encouraged and answered, and the doctor's availability to answer future questions firmly established.**

It is the eye doctor's professional and ethical responsibility to be thorough, knowledgeable, and caring, and to know her limits if there is some aspect of a given patient's care with which she is not totally familiar and comfortable. Consulting with a diabetic patient's other health care providers, or referring that patient to another eye doctor who has more experience with a particularly unusual or difficult problem, are not signs of inexperience, but of excellent professional judgment.

Types of Eye Doctors

There are several different types of eye doctors, a fact that is sometimes confusing to both patients and other health care professionals alike. This diversity is, in my view, advantageous for patients because each kind of eye care provider has unique strengths which, when used in a spirit of professional cooperation, combine to give all patients better care than the separate parts could on their own.

Here is a brief description of the various kinds of eye doctors:

Optometrist — Optometrists are, most often, the eye care equivalent of the family doctor. They are trained and licensed to *diagnose and treat disorders and diseases of the eyes and visual system through non-surgical means*, including the use of prescription eye drops (and oral medications in most states), as well as to detect the ocular manifestations of systemic disease (for example, diabetes) and refer patients to other health care specialists for eye surgery and/or further medical evaluation. Optometrists perform the majority of routine eye examinations in the United States.

Optometrists are not medical doctors (M.D. degree), but doctors of optometry (O.D. degree). Becoming an optometrist requires four years of pre-medical undergraduate education (identical to medical doctors) and then an additional four years of optometry school. Optometry school education consists of courses in geometric, physical and physiological optics, ocular anatomy and physiology, general anatomy and physiology, general and ocular pathology, general and ocular pharmacology, ocular manifestations of systemic disease, binocular vision, vision therapy, pediatric vision, geriatric vision, refraction, cosmetic and medical contact lens applications, and specialized electrodiagnostic testing.

The final two of four years is spent seeing patients in eye clinics and hospitals, including externships with eye surgeons and sub-specialists, and conducting original ophthalmic research. Three sets of national board examinations and individual state board examinations are required for licensure, with mandatory continuing education requirements every one to two years (depending upon the particular state). Some doctors of optometry complete an additional one-year residency, in areas such as ocular disease and low vision, and a few complete multi-year specialty fellowships in areas like retinal disease and glaucoma (see below).

Ophthalmologist — Ophthalmologists are medical doctors (M.D. degree) who *specialize in the medical and surgical treatment of eye disease,* as well as the ocular manifestations of systemic diseases (like diabetes). Like optometrists, ophthalmologists also see patients for routine eye care, including prescription of eyeglasses and contact lenses. The majority of ophthalmologists have completed a surgical residency and practice in affiliation with a hospital or ambulatory surgery center.

Becoming an ophthalmologist requires four years of premedical undergraduate education, four years of medical school, and an additional three to six years of residency training, depending upon the degree of sub-specialization. The medical school curriculum covers all aspects of human disease and principles of medical treatment and management, with only basic training in eye disease and the human visual system. Ophthalmology residency training focuses on diagnosis of eye disease, as well as medical, surgical and laser treatment of eye conditions.

As the surgical skills required for eye surgery are so demanding, a great deal of time is spent honing those skills. Ophthalmologists must pass rigorous national licensure examinations and a series of board examinations in order to practice. Continuing medical education requirements must be met for re-licensure. After ophthalmology residency, some doctors receive additional fellowship training in sub-specialties such as glaucoma, oculoplastics (eyelid and eye socket surgery), corneal disease and retinal disease.

Retina Specialist — Retina specialists are eye doctors, typically ophthalmologists*, who have completed additional sub-specialty fellowship training in the diagnosis and medical, surgical, and laser treatment of *retinal disease*. Other eye doctors, both optometrists and ophthalmologists, refer many of their patients to retina specialists, who frequently see the most complicated and challenging retinal diseases. A large percentage of retina specialty practices consist of patients with diabetic retinopathy.

Which is Best?

The "best" eye doctor for any particular patient depends upon that patient's unique needs and circumstances. For the average patient seeking a thorough, comprehensive eye examination, both optometrists and ophthalmologists do a fine job. For a diabetic with no previous history of diabetic eye disease, both types of doctors are again fine. For diabetics with diabetic eye disease *not* severe enough to require surgi-

---

* *Interestingly, some optometrists __do__ specialize in retinal disease. The largest and best retina specialty practice in the author's area has two fellowship-trained ophthalmologists and one fellowship trained optometrist on staff.*

cal or laser treatment, both optometrists and ophthalmologists are trained, licensed and qualified to follow those patients; both professionals have considerable training in and experience with the diagnosis and medical (non-surgical) treatment of diabetic eye disease, including retinopathy, glaucoma, keratopathy, and cranial neuropathy. For diabetics requiring *surgical treatment* of cataract or glaucoma, or laser treatment of retinopathy, an ophthalmologist experienced with these specific surgeries or treatments — *in diabetic patients* — is the best and only choice. For patients with severe or complicated retinopathy, or those requiring intra-ocular surgery to treat diabetic retinopathy, a retina specialist is undoubtedly the best choice.

A major advantage of this tiered system of eye doctors is that patients may be referred to specialists whose practice is limited to those patients' individual eye conditions (whether they have glaucoma, corneal disease, optic nerve disease, retinal disease, uveitis, or some other kind of eye disease, there is an ophthalmologic or optometric sub-specialist for that specific disease.)

As with any profession, some doctors, both optometrists and ophthalmologists, will have more knowledge, experience, and compassion than others will. **No matter which type of eye doctor a diabetic patient sees, the most important consideration is finding someone knowledgeable about and experienced with diabetic eye disease.** My recommendation is to ask your prospective eye doctor about her knowledge and experience, using this book as a guide.

Questions to Ask Your Eye Doctor

1. Do you have a lot of experience with diabetes and its various effects on the eyes?

2. Do you (or do other doctors in your practice) have any special interest in diabetic eye disease?

3. Do I have any signs of diabetic eye disease? Do I have any cataract, glaucoma, corneal problems, retina problems or eye muscle problems that are being caused by diabetes?

4. Has my eyeglass prescription changed significantly? If it has, is it likely caused by poor blood sugar control?

5. If I don't have any diabetic eye disease, when do you want to see me again?

6. If I do have diabetic eye disease, how do you recommend we manage or treat it? When do you want to check my condition again? Are you experienced with the surgical or laser treatment of diabetic eye disease? If my condition worsens, will you refer me to a sub-specialist?

7. Do you have any recommendations on how to avoid or reduce eye complications from diabetes?

8. Will you send a report of your diagnosis and recommendations to my other doctors? Would you like me to ask my diabetes doctor to send you a report of her findings and recommendations?

Chapter Fifteen:

Low Vision

Knowledge is Power, and a form of Cheap Insurance

Unfortunately, many people have already suffered the eye complications of diabetes. More tragically, many people will continue to suffer vision loss in spite of all we know, and the good news about prevention and effective treatments. Hopefully, far fewer diabetics will experience complications in the future. Hopefully, a definitive cure for diabetes is just "around the bend."

Until that time, though, it is very important that all diabetics know about what can be done, right now, to help them cope with vision loss.* For those who have already experienced vision loss, this chapter may serve as a primer on what's available and how to get started. For those who haven't lost vision from diabetes, the information in this chapter might best be viewed as an insurance policy of sorts; hopefully, it will never be needed, but it will be nice to have some familiarity with this material, "just in case."

---

*Again, I speak from painful, personal experience with temporary vision loss. After having pan-retinal laser photocoagulation for my proliferative diabetic retinopathy, I experienced vitreous hemorrhage in both of my eyes simultaneously. The blood cleared after about six months, but my vision was severely reduced (to about 20/400, with glasses) for the first four months; I was in graduate school, and could barely find my classes, much less read the required several hundred pages a day of course work. I didn't get, and was never offered, low vision services, but swore I would be better prepared for any future vision loss, for my own and my patients' sake, once I became an optometrist.

"Low Vision" refers to persons who have sub-normal vision from eye disease, *and* to the eye care specialty that helps those patients maximize whatever remaining visual potential they may have. There are many causes of low vision; the leading cause in the U.S. is macular degeneration (deterioration of the macula usually seen in older individuals), followed by glaucoma, and diabetic retinopathy. As discussed earlier in this book, diabetes is the leading cause of legal blindness (and hence, low vision) for younger Americans (ages 20-74). As different eye diseases affect vision in different ways, techniques for improving visual function vary considerably from disease to disease, as well as from patient to patient, but there are some general principles applying to all low vision care.

The goal of low vision care is to improve patients' visual functioning; that is, **to enable patients to engage in the day to day life tasks that give humans at least some autonomy and independence.** This may mean allowing a patient to read her mail or sign her name, correctly push numbers on a telephone or keys on a keyboard, cook and bathe without injuring herself, or utilize public transportation. **It does not mean that patients' vision is restored to what it was prior to the onset of eye disease, for that is not (yet) possible.** This last fact is terribly disconcerting to all low vision patients, but realization and acceptance of this fact are critical to the success of low vision treatment, which depends on active participation by the patient and a positive attitude. *Low vision care does not make it like it used to be, but it does make the most of what it is now.*

Low vision treatment is based upon two primary strategies: increasing **magnification**, and improving **contrast**. Let's take a very straightforward example of magnification. Suppose someone with diabetic retinopathy has experienced permanent vision loss; instead of having 20/20 visual acuity on the eye chart, he now has 20/200 acuity in his better seeing eye, and with the absolute best eyeglass prescription — he is, by definition, "legally blind." Having 20/200 acuity means that he can see from 20 feet away what somebody with normal eyesight can see from 200 feet away. Our hypothetical patient must be 10 times closer (200 / 20 = 10) to the eye chart to see the same size letters as a normally sighted person. How can he be helped to use his poorer vision more effectively?

Magnification

There are several ways, in fact. One is to **move closer physically to the thing he is trying to see**; if our patient can't read a street sign, let's say, from the same distance as his normally sighted friends, he can walk 10 times closer to the sign, at which point he *will* be able to read the sign. Moving closer magnifies the sign. **This way of magnifying things, by moving or holding them closer, is called "relative distance magnification,"** because we are enlarging them by changing their relative distance to us. The same principle applies to reading printed material (for example, books or magazines) up close. If our patient can't read words in a book from 16 inches away, he can hold the book much closer (ten times closer, or 1.6 inches from his eyes), with the help of specialized reading glasses that allow him to focus on those words at such a close distance.

Another way to magnify things is through the use of *telescopes, microscopes, and magnifiers*, devices which **"optically enlarge"** objects, just as an astronomical telescope magnifies distant heavenly bodies, or a microscope magnifies tiny bacteria. Low vision **telescopes** are used for sighting more distant things, like our hypothetical street sign, *without having to physically move closer to them*. These are typically hand held devices, and quite compact. Our visually impaired diabetic patient could carry this with him to read street signs

or wall-mounted menus, etc. Low vision **microscopes** magnify reading material *held at a more normal reading distance*,
and usually are mounted into a conventional pair of eyeglasses.
Our hypothetical patient with 20/200 vision from diabetic
retinopathy needs things magnified ten times in order to see
objects someone with 20/20 vision can identify, so he could
use a 10x power telescope to see the street sign, or a 10x
power microscope to read print up close.

Magnifying lenses of various strengths can be placed into
a hand held lens holder (just like a magnifying glass) or a
specially designed stand (called a stand magnifier), both of
which allow a more normal working distance (the distance
between the user's eyes and the object to be viewed.) A more
sophisticated method for optically magnifying near vision
materials (books, check registers, photographs, coins, you
name it) is use of a **closed circuit television video system**
(known as *CCTV*). CCTV devices feature a wide range of
magnification settings (a feature making them useful to patients with various degrees of visual impairment), reverse
polarity (black letters on a white background, or white letters
on a black background), and ample room for the user's hands
(allowing the user to sign documents or otherwise manipu-
late materials being viewed); some have a built-in display
screen, and some can be connected to a television set. The
primary disadvantage to CCTVs is their higher cost ($1,000
to $4,000) and bulk (although a few portable devices are now
available).

A third way of magnifying the world is by **physical enlargement**. Large numbers on a telephone touch pad, large
numbered clocks, and large print books or magazines are examples. Unfortunately, many forms of printed material are
not readily available in large print (a customer service-ori-
ented print shop or copy business is a good resource for getting print enlarged — this is how I got through my first se-
mester of graduate school with 20/400 vision.) Our hypo-

thetical patient with low vision could enlarge his reading material ten times or, alternatively, enlarge it five times in combination with an optical magnifier (like a hand held or stand magnifier) which provides another two times magnification (5x magnification times 2x magnification = 10x total magnification).

The amount of magnification any given patient needs depends upon a number of factors, all of which a low vision specialist can readily determine. In general, though, low vision patients don't necessarily need to see 20/20 size street signs or print in order to function. Typically, magnification sufficient to allow patients to recognize 20/40 size objects is quite adequate for most real world needs. This is accomplished by reducing the required magnification in the above examples by half; our hypothetical patient with 20/200 vision only needs five times magnification (5x) to see 20/40 size objects (200 / 40 = 5). Being five times closer to street signs or reading material can accomplish this, as can the use of optical aids (telescopes, microscopes, magnifiers) that produce 5x magnification, or physical enlargement of print by five times, or any combination of these techniques that yields a total of 5x magnification.

A drawback to all forms of magnification is that **these devices typically limit the user's field of view, the amount of the world, or number of words on a page, that can be viewed at any one time** (anyone who has ever used a pair of binoculars knows that you can't walk around while looking through them, because you will bump into objects not in your limited field of view.) This makes reading much slower than normal but, with practice and instruction from a low vision specialist, reading speed and ease of use do improve. Diabetic patients are often ideal candidates for many of these devices because many diabetics with vision loss are younger and, perhaps, more adaptable than at least some older patients.

Contrast Enhancement

Contrast enhancement makes objects of any given size easier to see by making those objects "stand out" more. Put another way, increasing contrast improves visual acuity independently of magnification (see Chapter 8, Figure 8.2 for an example of high and low contrast). **Among the ways of improving contrast are: improving lighting, improving print quality, enhancing the contrast between objects and the background which surrounds them, and use of colored filters over the eyes.** Brighter, closer incandescent lighting angled in such a way as to minimize reflections and glare often helps low vision patients to read more easily, as does darker and denser print on a light background; adhering dark colored materials at each edge of light colored stairs will make those steps more visible to a person with impaired vision; specially tinted eyeglass lenses will often enhance contrast between curbsides and the street when navigating outside of the home. These are just a few examples of how contrast enhancement might help patients with low vision due to diabetes or other conditions.

Adaptive Low Vision Products

A whole range of **adaptive products** are available for visually impaired and blind patients alike, including large print books and books on tape, large numbered and talking clocks, easy-to-thread sewing needles, large type and tactile stovetop knobs, specialized wood working tools, easy to fasten clothing items, and pill bottle magnifiers. The list goes on and on. For diabetics in particular, large display and talking blood glucose meters are available, as are syringe magnifiers and tactile insulin syringes that allow patients to accurately measure insulin dosages, even with no useful vision whatsoever.

Where Do I Find Low Vision Services?

Low vision specialists are, most often, optometrists and ophthalmologists. However, many dedicated non-eye doctors work closely with visually impaired patients, including mobility specialists, occupational counselors, and other specialists who teach even totally blind patients how to safely complete tasks of daily living like cooking, shaving, and taking prescription medications. Braille and guide dog services are also available for persons with extremely reduced or no vision. I have listed some excellent low vision resources (including web site addresses) at the end of this chapter. To find an eye doctor specializing in low vision in your area, you can start here or ask your own eye doctor for a referral.

Some metropolitan areas now have low vision centers with low vision specialists on staff, including eye doctors, and even a low vision store that allows patients and their families to try out various devices before purchasing them. Unfortunately, most insurance pays little or nothing for low vision services or products, so trying products before buying them is especially important. Equally important is receiving professional training on how to use these products, as research clearly shows that the more training low vision patients receive, the more likely they are to be successful with various visual aids.

A List of Useful Low Vision Organizations

Lighthouse International
111 East 59th Street
New York, NY 10022-1202
(800)-829-0500
www.lighthouse.org
   *an international clearinghouse for all aspects of low
   vision care and products*

**National Federation for the Blind -
Diabetes Action Network**
1412 I-70 Drive SW, Suite C
Columbia, MO 65203
(573) 875-8911
www.nfb.org/voice.htm
   *low vision services, including a catalog of large print,
   Braille and audiocassette material; publishes* Voice of
   the Diabetic, *an excellent newsletter on all aspects of
   diabetes*

Community Services for the Blind and Partially Sighted
9709 Third Avenue NE Suite 100
Seattle, WA 98115-2027
(800) 458-4888
www.csbps.org
   *regional low vision center with an excellent low vision
   catalog and store*

Low Vision Council
5921 South Middlefield Rd
Littleton, CO 80123
(303)797-6554
www.lowvisioncouncil.org
dedicated to education about low vision

American Council of the Blind
1155 15th Street NW
Suite 1004
Washington, D.C. 20005
(800) 424-8666
www.acb.org
*many services for the visually impaired, with an
emphasis on employment opportunities*

American Optometric Association
www.aoa.org/conditions/low_vision.asp
*information on low vision, eye disease and other
vision problems*

American Academy of Ophthalmology
www.eyenet.org
information on low vision and eye disease

<u>Key Points</u>

1. "Low Vision" refers to patients with reduced vision from eye disease, and to the specialty that works to help those patients maximize their remaining vision.

2. Low vision devices work by increasing magnification, contrast, or both.

3. A variety of low vision devices are available. Patients typically receive maximum benefit using several different kinds of devices, and with professional advice and instruction.

4. There is *always* something that can be done to help visually impaired or blind patients.

5. A significant percentage of people with low vision have diabetes. Understanding some low vision basics is like having insurance against diabetic eye disease.

Conclusion:

Living With Diabetes And Finding A Cure

I have written this book to help all diabetic patients and their families formulate a better strategy for living with diabetes and the health dangers it poses. The truth is, diabetes is a very serious medical condition, but it is something that each of us diabetics is capable of living with, and living well. Based on the mountain of diabetes research that has already been done, most experts believe that most diabetes complications can be avoided or reduced dramatically. As for diabetic eye disease, it is probable that 80% or more of all severe vision loss is preventable given the knowledge and treatments that are already available to our health care providers and us.

In reading hundreds of journal articles, position statements and editorials as I was preparing this text, I discovered more reason than ever for optimism about living with diabetes, as well as belief that a cure is only a matter of time and money dedicated to diabetes research. I also discovered a small but vocal minority of people who believe that too much research has focused on *living* with diabetes, on preventing its complications, rather than on finding a cure. The argument is sometimes made that preventative strategies, which emphasize improved glycemic control and lifestyle modification, place too much burden and **blame** on *diabetics themselves* for any complications that arise, rather than on the *disease* that causes so many complications. If individual diabetics lose vision, or kidney function, or suffer nerve damage or heart disease, it becomes their fault; we are, so this argument goes, blaming the victim rather than the disease.

I believe this position is misguided, because many of the scientific advancements in molecular biology, which *now* make a cure for diabetes a real possibility, were not available or even conceived of when major studies like the DCCT and UKPDS were started. Moreover, the techniques and treatments that will ultimately cure diabetes take time to develop, time that increases the risk of complications for patients who have diabetes *today* and who want, as any person would want, to minimize complications based upon the best scientific evidence. **There is no reason that we can't live well with diabetes *and* find a cure.**

This position does, however, underscore the importance of committing substantial resources to finding a cure (or cures) for a disease that causes so much suffering and has such a profound economic impact. Blaming individual diabetics for their own complications is not only unsympathetic and unproductive, but also erroneous, as a health care system that doesn't adequately educate and empower those individuals to reduce complications is also to blame. The problem is diabetes, not the people who are afflicted with it. The solution is knowledge, education, and eradication of diabetes, not blame. There are, no doubt, many scientific and political obstacles to overcome on route to a cure, but we must continue boldly and vigorously on that route.

A. Paul Chous, M.A., O.D.
Maple Valley, Washington

GLOSSARY

arteriosclerosis — refers to thickening and loss of elasticity in the arteries; hardening of the arteries

atherosclerosis — blockage of arteries by plaque, consisting of blood fats, proteins, complex carbohydrates and calcium

background diabetic retinopathy — small amounts of bleeding from damaged retinal capillaries, as well as deposits of blood proteins and fats within the retina; also called non-proliferative retinopathy

cataract — clouding of the eye's internal lens causing loss of vision

cells — the fundamental building blocks of all living tissues; receive nourishment (glucose) and oxygen from the blood stream; the entry of glucose into cells is controlled by insulin

cornea — the transparent covering at the front of the eye; focuses light on the retina

DCCT — "Diabetes Control and Complications Trial;" landmark study that showed the benefits of tight blood sugar control in Type 1 diabetics

diabetic eye disease — refers to those eye diseases that are more common in diabetic patients

Diabetic Retinopathy Study (DRS) — large clinical study that demonstrated the effectiveness of laser treatment for preventing blindness caused by proliferative diabetic retinopathy

dilation — in the eyes, this refers to enlarging the pupils with eye drops, allowing the eye doctor to see more of the internal eye

ETDRS — 'Early Treatment of Diabetic Retinopathy Study'; large clinical study that demonstrated the effectiveness of laser treatment for preventing vision loss due to diabetic macular edema

endocrine — refers to glands that produce hormones and secrete them into the circulatory system (bloodstream)

endocrinologist — a medical doctor specializing in the treatment of glandular diseases; diabetologists are endocrinologists who further specialize in the treatment of diabetes

glaucoma — chronic, progressive damage to the optic nerve resulting in permanent vision loss

glycemic — referring to blood sugar (blood glucose)

glycemic index — a measure of how quickly particular foods are converted into blood glucose

glycogen — hormone produced by the liver that raises blood glucose

glycosylated hemoglobin — a test which measures average blood sugar levels over the preceding 8-12 weeks. Also called glycohemoglobin and hemoglobin-A-1-c (HbA1c)

HDL — high-density lipoprotein; the good kind of cholesterol; often too low in diabetics

hyperglycemia — abnormally high blood sugar level

hyperinsulinemia — high levels of insulin in the blood stream

hypertension — high blood pressure

hypoglycemia — abnormally low blood sugar level

hypoxia — refers to inadequate oxygen supply, or body tissues receiving inadequate oxygen

incidence — the total number of new cases of a particular phenomenon (medical condition) in one year's time within a particular population of individuals

insulin — a hormone secreted by the pancreas which allows living tissue to absorb energy (in the form of glucose) from the foods we eat

insulin resistance — loss of the body's ability to use insulin

ischemia — lack of blood supply; poor circulation

islet cells — cells in the pancreas responsible for making insulin

keratopathy — any chronic disease of the cornea

LDL — low-density lipoprotein; the bad, plaque-forming kind of cholesterol

lens — clear structure inside the eye that allows us to change focus from far to near

low vision — reduced vision due to eye disease

microvascular — refers to the body's smallest blood vessels, such as those in the retina and kidney

macrovascular — refers to large blood vessels, such as those from the heart and leading to the brain

macula — the part of the retina that allows detailed, color vision

macular edema — swelling and deposit of blood lipids/protein in the macula, often causing vision loss

neovascularization — the growth of new blood vessels

nephropathy — kidney damage; both hyperglycemia and hypertension contribute to this condition

neuropathy — damage to nerves; can be caused by hyperglycemia and/or poor circulation and may affect normal sensation, movement and/or function

ophthalmologist — a medical doctor specializing in the medical and surgical treatment of eye disease

optic nerve — the nerve that connects the eyes to the brain

optometrist — an eye doctor specializing in the non-surgical treatment of eye conditions and diseases

PRP — "pan-retinal photocoagulation;" laser burns applied to the retina for the treatment of proliferative retinopathy and neovascular glaucoma

pathophysiology — the biochemical and cellular changes associated with a particular disease

prevalence — the total number of cases of a given phenomenon (medical condition) within a particular population of individuals

proliferative diabetic retinopathy (PDR) — growth of new, abnormal blood vessels on the surface of the retina and optic nerve which, if left untreated, can lead to blindness

retina — the delicate, light-sensitive film that lines the inside wall of the eye; connected to the optic nerve

retinal specialist — an eye doctor specializing in the diagnosis and treatment of retinal diseases

retinopathy — any sickness of the retina; the leading cause of blindness in diabetics

traction retinal detachment — retinal detachment caused by the formation of fibrous scar tissue connecting the retina and vitreous, as happens in proliferative diabetic retinopathy

triglycerides — a type of blood fat that is stored by the body and may promote atherosclerosis

Type 1 Diabetes — chronic hyperglycemia caused by total loss of the body's ability to produce insulin

Type 2 Diabetes — chronic hyperglycemia caused by a relative lack of insulin, insulin resistance, or both

UKPDS — "United Kingdom Prospective Diabetes Study;" landmark study showing the benefits of tight blood sugar and blood pressure control in Type 2 diabetics

visual field — refers to the amount and sensitivity of a person's peripheral vision

vitreous — the clear gelatin filling the majority of the internal eye

vitrectomy — surgical removal of the vitreous

INDEX

About the Author

Dr. Paul Chous completed his undergraduate education at Brown University and UC Irvine, where he was elected to **Phi Beta Kappa** *in 1985. He received his Master's Degree in 1986 and his Doctorate of Optometry in 1991, both with highest honors from UC Berkeley. Dr. Chous was selected as the* **Outstanding Graduating Optometrist** *in 1991. He has practiced for 12 years in Renton, Kent, Auburn and Tacoma, Washington with special emphasis on diabetic eye disease and diabetes education. Dr. Chous serves as a consultant to the* **American Diabetes Association***, which honored him with its distinguished* **Public Service Award** *in 1998. He lives in Maple Valley, WA with his wife, Dr. Elizabeth Chous, his son, Atticus, and three cats. Dr. Chous has been a Type 1 diabetic since 1968.*

Dr. Chous may be contacted via email at
dr.chous@diabeticeyes.com

The Diabetic Eye Disease website:
www.diabeticeyes.com

LaVergne, TN USA
04 April 2010
178123LV00002BA/298/A